A Sutcliffe
27th April '82
Dulwich, London SE22.

Ketoconazole in the Management
of Fungal Disease

Ketoconazole in the Management of Fungal Disease

edited by

H.B. Levine

editorial advisory group

E. Drouhet
R.J. Hay
H.E. Jones
Angela Restrepo

ADIS Press

New York · Tokyo · Sydney · Mexico · Auckland · Hong Kong

Ketoconazole in the Management of Fungal Disease

National Library of Australia
Cataloguing-in-Publication entry

Ketoconazole in the Management of Fungal Disease

Bibliography
Includes index
ISBN 0 909337 36 5

1. Mycoses. 2. Ketoconazole.
I. Levine, H.B.

616'.015

First printing

ADIS Press
404 Sydney Road, Balgowlah, NSW 2093, Australia

Editor

H.B. Levine
University of California, Berkeley, Chairman, Medical Microbiology Department, Naval Biosciences Laboratory, Oakland, California, USA

Contributors

M. Borgers and H. Van den Bossche
Department of Cell Biology, Janssen Pharmaceutica, Beerse, Belgium

R.J. Hay
Department of Medical Microbiology, London School of Hygiene and Tropical Medicine, London, England

R.C. Heel
Australasian Drug Information Services, Auckland, New Zealand

H.E. Jones
Department of Dermatology, Emory University School of Medicine, Atlanta, Georgia, USA

H.B. Levine
University of California, Berkeley, Medical Microbiology Department, Naval Biosciences Laboratory, Oakland, California, USA

Editorial advisory group

E. Drouhet
Department of Mycology, Pasteur Institute, Paris, France

R.J. Hay
Department of Medical Microbiology, London School of Hygiene and Tropical Medicine, London, England

H.E. Jones
Department of Dermatology, Emory University School of Medicine, Atlanta, Georgia, USA

Angela Restrepo
Corporación, de Investigaciones Biológicas, Hospital Pablo Tobón Uribe, Medellin, Colombia

Foreword

More than a decade has passed since Ajello (1970) likened the mycoses to an iceberg with 'its vast bulk . . . submerged in a murky sea of ignorance.' He was referring to the absence of precise figures to describe the world's medical mycological problems, both the deep and the superficial infections. Even today, most systemic fungal diseases are not classified as notifiable to governmental health services. Further, physicians often fail to report faithfully those that are notifiable. As an example, in its report to the Deputy Director, the California Ad Hoc Coccidioidomycosis Advisory Committee (1980) estimated that the true number of cases of coccidioidomycosis was '10 times greater, perhaps more' than the reported average yearly figure of 500. The State Epidemiologist estimated that the true figure could be up to 30 times higher.

If under reporting of a life-threatening notifiable mycosis is common in California, how conservative must be those estimates throughout the world of the serious mycoses that do not immediately endanger life.

Information that is available points to fungal and yeast diseases as a problem of staggering proportions. As early as the 1950's, Vanbreuseghem (1950), Marples (1950) and Gonzalez-Ochoa (1956) showed for three continents that pityriasis versicolor infections occur in half the population of tropical countries. Scalp ringworm remains a world-wide scourge. In the United States alone, Ajello (1970) estimated $25 millions (1970 dollars!) were spent annually on antiringworm treatments.

The subcutaneous mycoses plague Africa, Asia and South America. The latter continent additionally contends with a paracoccidioidomycosis rate conservatively estimated at between 0.4 and 0.8 per 100,000 (Mackinnon, 1972). No estimate can be made of the frequency of occurrence of candidosis in its various forms, nor for the numbers of cases of the emerging group of nosocomial, iatrogenic and opportunistic fungal and yeast diseases. The deep mycoses, even with the present reporting limitations, account for more than 100,000 cases annually in the three Americas.

Yet, until recently, concerted efforts to develop new antifungal therapies were not given high priority by pharmaceutical houses. Clinicians and patients coped with mycological disease by relying upon half a dozen drugs which, especially for the systemic mycoses, were often of limited value or unacceptable toxicity. A change was to follow the discovery in 1944 that benzimidazole had antimycotic activities (Woolley, 1944). During the subsequent 35 years the therapeutic efficacy of substituted imidazoles in fungal disease was explored by many, most notably Janssen Pharmaceutica. The trail led to ketoconazole, a broad-spectrum, orally-active antimycotic with few and minimal side effects.

The spectrum of ketoconazole's antimicrobial activities is covered in this book. The editors have taken care to point out the limitations of the drug. Much of the information has been drawn from clinical studies by 120 investigators from 20 countries for which a common protocol was used. This provided for standardised clinical and microbial criteria for inclusion, assessment, and analysis of results. A standardised approach has also been adopted to reporting the results of these studies; in particular, even small raised lesions with no evidence of active disease and with negative microbiological results, have been classified as 'marked improvement' rather than 'remission'. As often happens in the early clinical trials of new drugs, many of the patients studied provided an especially stringent test of the efficacy of ketoconazole as their fungal infections were of longstanding or had proved resistant to other therapies. The studies are, as yet, largely unpublished but have been documented and submitted to the United States Food and Drug Administration, the Canadian Health Protection Branch and the Australian Health Department in support of new drug applications for ketoconazole.

This volume is an in-depth review of ketoconazole. It deals with all aspects of the drug — its influence on the dermatomycoses, on candidosis of the mouth and vagina, on systemic and chronic mucocutaneous candidosis and on candiduria. It summarises current information on ketoconazole therapy of the deep and the percutaneous mycoses, histoplasmosis, coccidioidomycosis, paracoccidioidomycosis and chromomycosis. Other chapters describe the drug's mechanism of action, its pharmacokinetics and its metabolism. It is, in short, a handbook.

H.B. Levine, Ph.D.
Oakland, California

References

Ajello, L.: The medical mycological iceberg. Proceedings of the International Symposium on the Mycoses. p.3-12 (Pan American Health Organisation, Washington, DC 1970).

California Ad Hoc Coccidioidomycosis Advisory Committee: Report to the Director, State Health Services (1980).

Gonzalez-Ochoa, A.: Pityriasis versicolor. Revista Médica (Mex) 2: 81 (1956).

Mackinnon, J.E.: Geographic distribution and prevalence of paracoccidioidomycosis. Proceedings First Pan American Symposium on Paracoccidioidomycosis, Medellin, Colombia: 45 (1972).

Marples, M.J.: The incidence of certain skin diseases in Western Samoa; a preliminary survey. Transactions Royal Society of Tropical Medicine and Hygiene, 44: 319 (1950).

Vanbreuseghem, R.: Un problème de mycologie médicale; le pityriasis versicolor. Annales Institut Pasteur (Paris) 79: 798 (1950).

Woolley, D.W.: Some biological effects produced by benzimidazole and their reversal by purines. Journal of Biological Chemistry 152: 225 (1944).

Editor's Note

Much of the unpublished information on which this book is based is held in the Janssen Research Foundation, Beerse, Belgium. We felt the constant repetition of 'on file at the Janssen Research Foundation' might become wearisome for our readers and have only used this attribution selectively. Where a statement is not otherwise referenced it may be assumed that it is based on data from this source.

In the multicentre clinical studies reported here a common definition of 'remission' and 'marked improvement' was adopted. This was:

Remission: Negative mycological culture and other direct or indirect evidence of mycotic infection (e.g. microscopy, serology) after treatment and disappearance of all clinical evidence of disease.

Marked improvement: Persistence of small residual lesions only, without evidence of active disease.

In many instances patients who were categorised as markedly improved at the time the data was analysed had not completed their course of treatment.

H.B. Levine

Acknowledgements

Without the encouragement and interest of Dr Paul Janssen and Mr Jim Bodine, and the support of the Janssen Research Foundation, this book could never have been written. The authors are also indebted to the clinical investigators whose studies of ketoconazole gave rise to so much of the data on which this account of the drug is based:

R. Galimberti, R. Negroni, G. Weisburd, *Argentina;* J. Aussems, H. Baes, S. Bataille, H. Campaert, P. Coolen-Cryns, J. Daubresse, J. De Bersaques, J. Debois, J. Decroix, F. Delbrouck-Poot, J. Delescluse, M. De Lune, P. De Munck, F. Dethier, J. Devriendt, J. De Weert, J. Dhont, P. Dockx, F. Fierens, M. Geerts, D. Gielen-Mathus, J. Halloy-Robience, C. Henry, R. Hols, L. Huwarts, J. Lambert, A. Legrain, R. Lerut, F. Maes, R. Mertens, J. Morias, J. Oleffe, D. Parent, W. Peremans, G. Pierard, J. Pierard, C. Pirard, D. Platevoet, J. Porters, E. Rollier, L. Rutgeerts, F. Schreer, D. Tennstedt, M. Thulliez, L. Van Lint, D. Van Neste, L. Verhoeve, J. Vertommen, W. Wellens, R. 'T Kint, *Belgium;* R. Baruzzi, L. Cuce, G. Del Negro, *Brazil;* A. Restrepo, *Colombia;* J. Erben, M. Horcicka, B. Sukova, B. Vach, *Czechoslovakia;* E. Svejgaard, *Denmark;* F. Desmons, B. Echenne, B. Kalis, *France;* H. Grimmer, E. Haneke, D. Konietzko, J. Tofahrn, G. Zamfirescu, *Germany;* J. Bran, *Guatemala;* I. Herjavecz, I. Torok, *Hungary;* B. Callaghan, *Ireland;* R. Chacore, A. Norma, S. Sarabia, A. Saul, O. Welsh, *Mexico;* E. Heid, *Morocco;* J. Groen, J. Keuning, A. Reuling, *Netherlands;* J. Morrison, *South Africa;* A. Aliaga Donice, R. Castells, R. Montserrat, J. Vilate, *Spain;* J. Zellweger, *Switzerland;* R. Hay, D. Oakley, *UK;* R. Alford, R. Barbee, A. Catanzaro, A. Daily, J. Fields, C. Foster, J. Galgiani, R. Glogau, J. Graybill, J. Hanifin, P. Hermans, M. Hilty, S. Horowitz, H. Jones, C. Kirkpatrick, I. Krupp, S. Levin, H. Levine, R. Libke, H. Lischner, R. Owen, I. Rex, T. Slama, E. Smithwick, D. Stevens, E. Stiehm, N. Zaias, *USA;* D. Borelli, *Venezuela:*

to those who, with the general coordinator Dr Jan Symoens, supported and monitored these studies in the various countries:

E. Scharenberg, *Argentina;* H. Longueville, M. Mourlon-Beernaert, B. Nuyten, J. Polak, A. Reyntjens, H. Scheijgrond, *Benelux;* W. de Oliveira Neto, *Brasil;* F. Hansen, *Denmark;* J.M. Lecomte, *France;* P. Oettel, *Germany;* R. Alcantara, *Mexico;* A. Bartlett, *Spain;* M. Emanuel, *UK;* J. Brugmans, B. Legendre, *USA:*

and finally to:

J. Heeres, J. Van Cutsem, M. De Brabander, J. Heykants and R. Marsboom for their contribution to preclinical studies and T. Aerts, Annie Baisier, J. Dom, Maria Elst, C. Hörig, M. Moens, J. Peeters, R. Rutten, S. Van Gestel and R. Vermeer

who were involved in the retrieval, checking, tabulation, statistical analysis, art presentation and initial technical reporting of the data under the central coordination of Viviane Schuermans.

Contents

Mycoses and Antimycotics

Chapter I

Superficial and Deep Mycoses: The Extent of the Problem

R.J. Hay

There are a great number of human diseases which can be attributed in some way to the effects of fungi. Their influence may be indirect, for instance by their contribution to the destruction of foodstuffs, or may depend on their toxic or antigenic properties. Alternatively fungi may cause disease by invasion of tissue. Such infections caused by fungi, the mycoses, have long been recognised as important, but not necessarily common, problems in all spheres of medicine.

The Superficial Mycoses

Superficial infections caused by fungi include some of the commonest of cutaneous diseases such as pityriasis versicolor as well as the most resistant to therapy, chronic mucocutaneous candidosis (table I).

The Dermatophytes

Dermatophyte infections are caused by fungi which invade the keratinised zones of epidermis as well as hair and nail. These infections are common and may be difficult to treat, although diagnosis rarely presents problems. Amongst the clinical patterns of infection produced by the dermatophytes are athletes foot, scalp ringworm and onychomycosis. Although the types of infection and their presentation have not changed over recent years the causative organisms have, and a major feature has been the rise to prominence over the last 40 years of *Trichophyton rubrum*. At the beginning of this century infections in Europe and the USA caused by *T. rubrum* were sufficiently unusual to merit reporting in the dermatological literature. The situation has now changed, so that in a dermatological clinic *T. rubrum* infections may account for 75% or more of culturally proven dermatophyte infections. The presumed spread of the organism from the Far East has largely taken place since World War II (Hildick-Smith et al., 1964). The importance of *T. rubrum* to a clinician is its resistance to therapy. The organism occupies a secure ecological niche, commonly the epidermis of the soles and toe web spaces as well as nail keratin, from which it is difficult to dislodge. Infections are often characterised by lack of inflammation and by chronicity. T lymphocyte mediated responses, which are important in limiting dermatophyte infections, may be weak and ineffective in chronic *T. rubrum* infections (Hanifin et al., 1974). Similar poor responses may occur in patients whose infections respond to therapy, suggesting that the organism *per se* is associated with immunological hyporeactivity depending on the clinical site of infection (Hay and Brostoff, 1977).

Scalp ringworm: Endemic scalp ringworm, once common in school children, has been effectively controlled in many parts of the world through the widespread use of drugs such as griseofulvin (Grin, 1962). In these areas its place has been taken by scalp infections caused by zoophilic organisms such as *Microsporum canis* derived from the cat or dog. Infections caused by such organisms are sporadic or occur in small outbreaks. However despite effective drug therapy the prevalence of scalp ringworm caused by these dermatophytes remains relatively constant. The presence of a reservoir of infection and asymptomatic carriage by domestic animals is largely responsible. This situation is not uniform throughout the world and in many countries, particularly Africa, endemic scalp infection caused by anthropophilic dermatophytes, spread from man to man, such as *M. audouinii*, remains a major problem (Soyinka, 1979). The exact extent of the problem remains a matter for speculation and its resolution depends on the acquisition of accurate epidemiological data and subsequent control measures.

Table I. Human superficial mycoses

Clinical manifestation	Causative organism
1. Mycoses of hair and scalp	
Tinea capitis	Dermatophytes
Favus	Dermatophytes
Black piedra	*Piedraia hortae*
White piedra	*Trichosporon cutaneum beigelii*
Trichomycosis axillaris[1]	*Corynebacterium tenuis*
2. Mycoses of the skin	
Dermatomycosis	Dermatophytes, yeasts
Tinea imbricata (Tokelau)	*Trichophyton concentricum*
Erythrasma[1]	*Corynebacterium minutissimum*
Pityriasis versicolor	*Malassezia furfur (Pityrosporum orbiculare)*
Tinea nigra	*Exophiala werneckii*
3. Mycoses of the nail	
Onychomycosis	Dermatophytes, yeasts
Perionyxis	Yeasts
4. Mycoses of the mucous membranes	
Oral thrush	*Candida albicans*
Vaginal candidosis	Candida and other yeasts
Gastrointestinal candidosis	Candida and other yeasts
5. Mucocutaneous mycoses	
Chronic mucocutaneous candidosis	*Candida albicans*

1 At present usually considered bacterial infections.

Tinea pedis: This is a common condition and in occupational groups and communities such as boarding schools it may reach epidemic proportions. Foot infections in coal miners, for instance, remain a major problem of occupational health (Gentles and Holmes, 1957). The commonest infecting organisms are *T. interdigitale* and *T. rubrum* and the high rate of infection has been associated with both the increased opportunity for spread of the organism, for instance in shower rooms, and working conditions which provide the ideal environment for the initiation of infection. Measures designed to control the former have included the removal of wooden 'duck' boards from shower units, regular foot inspections and issues of bathroom footwear, but the problem remains. Endemic tinea pedis in industry is not confined to coal miners but may occur in any occupational group, paticularly those where communal showering occurs or where working conditions or protective clothing enhance the chances of an infection occurring following exposure to the organism.

Vaginal Candidosis —
A Modern Epidemic

Superficial infections caused by *Candida* species are common. Likewise carriage of *Candida* by normal subjects is common. The risk of acquiring *Candida* is increased in a hospital environment (Jennison, 1977) and the incidence of carriage, for instance, rises during a hospital admission. However the acquisition of a *Candida* infection is not necessarily related to admission to hospital. A major problem of recent years has been the dramatic rise in the incidence of vaginal candidosis (Hurley and deLouvois, 1979). For instance a large London clinic for genitourinary medicine might see approximately 2,000 new cases of vaginal candidosis per year. Vaginal candidal infections have been associated with a number of factors most notably diabetes mellitus and pregnancy. However the enormous increase in the incidence of the infection cannot possibly be explained in terms of these factors alone. The contraceptive pill and increased sexual activity have also been held to be responsible, without adequate evidence. Other potential underlying factors include the possible predisposing role of other genital infections caused by organisms such as Chlamydia or Corynebacteria, asymptomatic carriage by males and changes of vaginal pH.

Although the high incidence of vaginal candidosis itself is a sufficient problem, it has become clear that recurrent and even chronic infections are common (Hurley and deLouvois, 1979). However there is no evidence that the failure of drugs to eradicate the infection is related to drug resistance and the predisposing factors in vaginal candidosis are almost certainly contributory to treatment failure. A solution to the problem would seem to depend on a closer understanding of these factors.

Hendersonula and Scytalidium

Amongst infections of palmar or plantar skin or nails, there are a group of superficial fungal infections caused by non-dermatophytes which bear a close clinical resemblance to the 'dry' type of infections caused by *T. rubrum*. The two organisms concerned are *Hendersonula toruloidea* and *Scytalidium hyalinum*. Although infected individuals have usually come from tropical areas such as the Caribbean, Africa, India or the Far East, the diagnosis is often made outside the patient's country of origin. The causative organisms in the environment are saprophytes or parasites, *Hendersonula,* for instance, being an important plant pathogen. The infections are not uncommon and in one clinic over a third of microscopically positive 'dermatophyte-like' infections in patients originating from the tropics were caused by *Hendersonula* or *Scytalidium* or both (Moore, 1978). A further feature of these organisms is that they fail to grow on laboratory media containing cycloheximide and they are also clinically resistant to all current therapy.

The Subcutaneous Mycoses

Mycetoma

Subcutaneous infections caused by fungi are not common, but assume undue clinical importance because of their chronicity, potential for local destruction and in some cases resistance to chemotherapy. Mycetoma (Madura foot) exemplifies the problem. This mycosis, a chronic infection of subcutaneous tissue and adjacent bone or skin, is characterised by the presence of aggregates of the causative fungi or actinomycete filaments, 'grains' (Mahgoub and Murray, 1973). Grains discharged from sinus openings are often not viable on laboratory isolation. However they form relatively indestructible foreign bodies in tissue, particularly when, as in the case of *Madurella mycetomi,* the outer layer of the grain is permeated with melanin-containing cement (Findlay and Vismer, 1974). Once this stage is reached destruction of the organism by drugs whose diffusion is hampered by the presence of pus may not disrupt the grain in any way, and the latter will continue to attract the inflammatory reaction responsible for the formation of sinuses. The infection is not common and is largely confined to tropical countries. In a clinic in the Sudan, for instance, approximately 200 new cases may be seen each year (Mahgoub and Murray, 1973) and in a worldwide survey in 1963 Mariat (Mariat, 1963) obtained information on 854 cases recorded over 20 years. None-the-less the importance of mycetoma lies in its chronicity and morbidity with the subsequent implications for both the patient himself and the local resources for health care.

Table II. The deep mycoses

Clinical manifestation	Causative organism
1. Subcutaneous mycoses	
Eumycotic mycetoma (maduromycosis)	
yellowish-white granules	*Petriellidium boydii, Acremonium* sp.
black granules	*Madurella* spp., *Exophiala jeanselmei*
Actinomycotic mycetoma[1]	
yellowish-white granules	*Actinomycetes*
Chromomycosis (dermatitis verrucosa)	*Phialophora* spp., *Fonsecea* spp.,
	Cladosporium carrionii
Sporotrichosis	*Sporothrix schenckii*
Lobomycosis (keloid blastomycosis)	*Loboa loboi*
Rhinosporidiosis	*Rhinosporidium seeberi*
2. Systemic mycoses	
Caused by yeasts	
Systemic candidosis	*Candida* spp.
Cryptococcosis (torulosis)	*Cryptococcus neoformans*
Geotrichosis	*Geotrichum candidum*
Torulopsidosis	*Torulopsis glabrata*
Caused by mold fungi	
Aspergillosis	*Aspergillus* spp.
Aspergilloma	*Aspergillus* spp.
Phycomycosis (mucormycosis)	*Rhizopus* sp., *Mucor* sp., *Basidiobolus* sp.
	Conidiobolus sp., *Absidia* sp.
Caused by actinomycetes	
Actinomycosis[1]	*Actinomyces* spp.
Nocardiosis[1]	*Nocardia asteroides*
Caused by dimorphic fungi	
Paracoccidioidomycosis	*Paracoccidioides brasiliensis*
Blastomycosis (North American-)	*Blastomyces dermatitidis*
Histoplasmosis	*Histoplasma capsulatum*
African histoplasmosis	*Histoplasma capsulatum* var. *duboisii*
Coccidioidomycosis (valley fever)	*Coccidioides immitis*

1   At present usually considered bacterial infections.

Drug treatment of mycetomas caused by actinomycetes is usually effective provided it is instituted at an early stage (Mahgoub, 1976). By contrast surgery is the treatment of choice in true fungal mycetomas, eumycetomas. In long established cases of actinomycetoma which fail to respond to therapy immune defects of T lymphocyte function may occur. From the foregoing it can be seen that early recognition of mycetoma may have a critical influence on the outcome of the infection. Unfortunately in endemic areas attempts to institute some form of surveillance have been severely curtailed by the distances and terrain involved and the financial implications. In addition fear of amputation, a common and necessary recourse in many cases, will prevent the local populace from presenting for early treatment.

Phaeohyphomycosis

Other subcutaneous infections present similar problems of diagnosis and management. Subcutaneous cystic infections (phaeohyphomycosis) caused by dematiacious, brown pigmented, fungi are being recognised with increased frequency. This group of subcutaneous infections has been diagnosed with increasing frequency in both temperate and tropical areas (Ichinose, 1971). In addition they have been seen in immunosuppressed patients and it is this particular group of patients which probably accounts for the increased reporting of the condition in recent years.

Opportunism and Systemic Fungal Infection

Systemic fungal infections in predisposed or immunocompromised individuals, the opportunistic mycoses, have increased enormously over the last 30 years. The rise in incidence has followed a number of significant medical advances, in particular the use of organ transplantation, improvements in the treatment of cancer and prolonged intravenous feeding. However it is clear that detailed information on the number of cases recognised is strictly limited by the effectiveness of current diagnostic methods and by the ability to confirm the cause of death by post-mortem examination (Baker, 1962).

Isolation of Organisms

The isolation of organisms such as *Candida* from systemically infected patients is successful in only a small proportion of genuine cases (Mirsky and Cuttner, 1972). In invasive aspergillosis and zygomycete infections (mucormycosis) the frequency of positive cultural isolations is even lower (Krick and Remington, 1976). Conversely a positive isolation of a potential opportunist must be examined critically in the light of clinical and radiological findings. For instance the presence of *Candida* in the sputum of an immunosuppressed patient may reflect oral or bronchial colonisation rather than invasive pulmonary candidosis, proven cases of which are rare. Likewise the isolation of Aspergilli from such patients must be treated circumspectly although *Aspergillus* species are not commonly isolated from patients' sputum apart from those with chronic pulmonary disease.

Serodiagnosis

Care must also be taken in the interpretation of serological findings (Krick and Remington, 1976). For instance detection of circulating antibody in cases of systemic *Candida* infection is extremely helpful, particularly in cases of endocarditis. However, even with the most accurate procedures, a small proportion of true cases of systemic candidosis escape serological detection (Kozinn et al., 1978). With invasive aspergillosis in immunosuppressed patients the proportion of serologically negative cases is higher, although with serial estimations and laboratory procedures with improved sensitivity a larger number of real cases of infection may be recognised. The detection of antigen in serum and body fluids has been used for some time in the detection of cryptococcal polysaccharide (Gordon and Vedder, 1966). The latex particle agglutination test or its variants such as the charcoal method have used inert particles coated with specific antiserum to measure the concentration of cryptococcal polysaccharide. Such methods have been highly successful, giving positive results in up to 95% of cases. The methods also have great value in assessing the prognosis and the effectiveness of treatment. However in *Candida* and *Aspergillus* infections serodiagnosis by measurement of antigen has been less successful. In the case of systemic candidosis it is likely that the formation of immune complexes starts to occur early in the infection and these may have to be separated into constituent antigen and antibody before immunological methods can be used for antigen detection (Segal et al., 1979). Techniques used to split complexes and the subsequent purification process are, of necessity, time consuming. Of more potential value is the use of gas liquid chromatographic analysis of serum from infected patients. The presence of certain by-products of *Candida*, particularly cell wall mannan, is diagnostic and these have been detected in genuine cases of systemic infection (Miller et al., 1974). However, so far this method has not been widely used.

Clinical Diagnosis

The diagnosis of systemic mycoses caused by opportunistic fungi can rarely be made on clinical grounds alone. One exception is the presence of the characteristic retinal lesions of candidosis (Fishman et al., 1972).

These are most often seen in *Candida* infections occurring in patients who are receiving prolonged intravenous feeding. They appear to be less common in patients with other varieties of systemic candidosis, although their presence should certainly be sought.

Histological Diagnosis

The most reliable method of laboratory diagnosis in this group of infections is histology, although the risks attendant in biopsying patients, particularly those with thrombocytopenia, may be great. Radiological abnormalities in the immunocompromised patient with an undiagnosed fever are common, and all too often nonspecific (Rosenbaum et al., 1974). Attempts to biopsy areas of radiological opacity have been very successful and in many instances have produced a diagnosis, although the frequency of complications has varied with the clinical state of the patient and the skill and experience of the operator. Various techniques are available and these range from transthoracic aspiration of x-ray opacities to per endoscopic bronchial biopsy (Krick and Remington, 1976). In each there is a definite risk of haemorrhage or pneumothorax. In many cases, open lung biopsy has proved to be the most reliable method although it carries the disadvantages of open chest surgery and anaesthesia.

Prevalence of Infection

The problems of diagnosis in systemic fungal infections are compounded by the deficiencies in our knowledge of the prevalence of each. It is very clear that, if post mortem data are compared with ante mortem diagnoses, systemic mycoses are grossly underdiagnosed particularly in patients with underlying leukaemia (Baker, 1962). However the opposite may be true. For instance proven cases of pulmonary candidosis in which invasion of lung parenchyma occurs are few. In one recent report this low incidence of histologically proven pulmonary infections caused by *Candida*, has been confirmed (Masur et al., 1978) and in many instances such invasion may occur following terminal aspiration of gastrointestinal contents. The number of cases of proven invasion is far outweighed by those patients at risk who are treated for pulmonary candidosis on the basis of a positive sputum culture. It should not be inferred from this that such patients should not be treated but only that it highlights deficiencies in our present methods of diagnosis and in the determination of the significance of results. A further example is the immunocompromised patient with a positive *Candida* blood culture. In many such patients removal of predisposing factors such as a central venous line may be associated with disappearance of the organism from blood without further therapeutic measures. However there is a risk, which is likely to be increased in patients with impaired immune responses, that either a metastatic focus of infection has been established prior to removal of the line or that an infection is left at the drip site (Krick and Remington, 1976). In such cases treatment is often given, but the significance of a clinical improvement is difficult to assess unless the extent of the infection can be clearly shown. The patient improves but the value of the drug is unknown. This makes the clinical assessment of new antifungal agents an extremely difficult task unless standardised criteria for such assessment are agreed.

It is also not clear to what extent patterns of infection by fungi vary between individual centres. The incidence of, for instance, invasive aspergillosis, may depend on environmental factors (Burton et al., 1972) particularly procedures used for ventilation of wards or side rooms. Cases of mucormycosis have been seen after use of contaminated dressing packs

(Gartenberg et al., 1978). A further unknown factor is the policy of each medical or surgical team towards immunosuppressive regimens or anti-tumour agents. It is likely that considerable variation in the incidence of infections which follow, for instance, neutropenia or immunosuppression, is likely in different centres when different regimens are employed. There are no published comparisons of such factors and indeed they would be difficult to compile. None-the-less it may be inaccurate to use statistics gathered from hospital A to assess the likely prevalence of fungal disease in hospital B even if the conditions being treated are similar in each centre.

In the last 20 years techniques of organ transplantation have changed considerably. Heart transplants are still attended by a significant risk of systemic fungal infection. However, in the field of renal transplantation there have been some improvements. In particular the numbers of cases of opportunistic infections has fallen in many units. Several factors have been responsible for this including the modification of immunosuppressive regimens. The use of prolonged and recurrent courses of drugs to treat rejection episodes has been revised and the patients' chances of survival have improved. Such measures are not so practicable in the case of heart transplants. The practice of bone marrow transplantation in patients with leukaemia or primary bone marrow disorders has become much more widespread in recent years. These patients are susceptible to both systemic and deep focal mycoses, in particular oesophageal candidosis. Although accurate figures for this group of patients are not available they would certainly show a significant incidence of opportunistic fungal infection.

Fungal infections in compromised patients remain a significant problem. In particular their prevalence, the variation between hospital centres and the methods of assessment of the extent of infection before treatment are areas where considerable improvement in our current knowledge would be greatly valued. In particular better methods of diagnosis are of the utmost importance.

Cryptococcosis — A Special Case

Cryptococcosis remains a special case amongst the systemic mycoses. In certain parts of the world infections occur predominantly in the compromised host. In the United Kingdom 93% of all cases of cryptococcosis notified to the Mycological Reference Laboratory, London, between 1970 and 1980 have occurred in patients with underlying disease, commonly sarcoidosis, Hodgkin's disease and collagen disorders such as systemic lupus erythematosus (Hay et al., 1980). By contrast, significant numbers of cases reported from elsewhere including the USA (Spickard et al., 1963) and Australia occur in patients with no underlying abnormality. Whether this reflects a difference in the nature of the organism or its distribution in the environment is unknown. However, it means that it is unreliable to compare the relative merits of diagnostic methods and treatment in different parts of the world unless the condition and influence of the host are considered. Whatever these differences there have been reports from many centres that more cases of cryptococcosis in man are being seen in recent years. It is not clear whether this reflects a genuine upsurge in the disease or increased recognition. Furthermore the incidence of the infection is likely to be much higher than expected if a substantial proportion of the population is sensitised to the organism following a subclinical infection. Subclinical infection in cryptococcosis is a likely possibility in the light of a number of findings. Experimental cryptococcosis can be regularly established in mice following inhalation of small numbers of yeast cells (Larsh et al., 1978) and the organism may be present in the environment, even in densely populated areas, in high concentrations. *Cryptococcus* can be isolated from sputum of asymptomatic individuals and pulmonary cryptococcosis may be an acute self limiting infection (Campbell, 1966). The ideal method of confirming the existence of subclinical cryptococcosis is with skin test surveys. Unfortunately no standard reagent is available although a number of preparations have been investigated. Preliminary work with some cryptococcal antigens confirms that a significant proportion of normal populations, including individuals selected at random and those who may be occupationally exposed to the organism (pigeon breeders), have positive delayed type hypersensitivity to the organism (Newberry et al., 1967). If such findings are confirmed, exposure to and subclinical infection caused by *Cryptococcus* is likely to be more widespread than originally thought.

Systemic Infections Caused by Pathogenic Fungi

Epidemiology

Epidemiological surveys and, in particular, skin testing have long since indicated the extent and prevalence of subclinical illness caused by the systemic mycoses which follow infection by pathogenic fungi such as *Histoplasma capsulatum* and *Coccidioides immitis* (Palmer et al., 1957). In these conditions the route of infection is almost always respiratory and the vast majority of those who inhale the organism develop a positive intradermal test if not actual symptoms of infection. Resolution without sequelae is the normal course of events. The evidence that wide subclinical exposure occurs in the other mycoses is less clear. In the case of blastomycosis there is no standardised skin test antigen. However in paracoccidioidomycosis, South American blastomycosis, some degree of subclinical infection seems likely in the light of skin test findings (Restrepo et al., 1968). Even in blastomycosis there have been a number of reports of acute self-limiting pulmonary blastomycosis in groups of individuals (Sarosi et al., 1974). Others exposed to the infection may develop asymptomatic radiological or serological changes. Unfortunately the sources of *Blastomyces dermatitidis* and *Paracoccidioides brasiliensis* in the environment are not clear.

With all the systemic mycoses within this group significant morbidity has been associated with laboratory exposure following either implantation or inhalation of an organism. This may limit the role of routine diagnostic laboratories unless appropriate facilities for isolation and containment of suspect cultures are available. A welcome advance which has gone much of the way towards solving this problem has been a method of detecting soluble antigens which diffuse from a culture 'in vitro' into an overlying aqueous layer (Standard and Kaufman, 1977). The latter is concentrated and antigen present detected serologically against standard antisera. This exoantigen method of identification of potentially dangerous cultures has considerably reduced the risk of laboratory acquired infection from such sources.

The Compromised Host

The systemic mycoses can and do occur in compromised individuals and it is only recently that the clinical pattern of disease has been shown to be affected by such factors. Chronic pulmonary histoplasmosis, for instance, is associated with both smoking and pulmonary emphysema (Goodwin et al., 1976). Rapidly disseminating histoplasmosis may occur in patients with lymphoma (Kauffman et al., 1978) and diabetics are prone to develop a progressive pulmonary form of coccidioidomycosis (Drutz and Cantanzaro, 1978b). Serious forms of these disorders are also associated with the immunosuppressive drugs given with renal or cardiac transplants. The underlying condition of the host is therefore of considerable importance in determining not only the pattern of infection but also its course and prognosis. Ultimately the success of therapy will depend on such factors.

It has also been recognised that defects of immune function may be seen in mycoses caused by the systemic pathogens. Anergy to intradermal coccidioidin often accompanies disseminated forms of coccidioidomycosis and *in vitro* T lymphocyte hyporeactivity may occur (Drutz and Cantanzaro, 1978a). Similarly defective lymphocyte transformation has been seen in disseminated histoplasmosis (Cox, 1979). B lymphocyte function in such cases appears to be intact and high titres of antibody may indicate established dissemination. However in chronic infections the pattern of immunoglobulin production may change, high levels of IgE, for instance, being found (Cox and Arnold, 1980). These findings indicate profound changes in immune function occurring during infections with systemic pathogens such as *Histoplasma*. Although some such defects may antedate the onset of the infection, others may follow it. Treatment with chemotherapy or transfer factor in patients with coccidioidomycosis may reverse cutaneous anergy to intradermal antigen (Cantanzaro et al., 1974). There is evidence in histoplasmosis that secondary T lymphocyte hypofunction may follow recruitment of suppressor lymphocytes (Stobo et al., 1976). Other methods of immune modulation such as disruption of T lymphocyte recirculation and histamine mediated T cell suppression secondary to an infective process are not well understood. However, defective host resistance whatever its cause has undoubtedly contributed significantly to chemotherapeutic failures and chronicity in the systemic mycoses.

The Reporting of Mycoses

Accurate statistics on incidence, morbidity and distribution of mycoses are limited by the fact that fungal infections are not notifiable conditions. Data is therefore gathered by voluntary contributions of information to certain major centres or laboratories which in turn attempt to process material received. Some of the difficulties attendant in the reporting of mycoses have been outlined. They include the presence of large numbers of subclinical infections in certain mycoses which may be highly significant. For instance it has been calculated on the basis of skin test conversions that approximately 5×10^5 individuals are infected by *H. capsulatum* in the USA each year (Furcolow, 1957). With the opportunistic fungi accurate estimates of the prevalence of infection depend on widescale post mortem data which is rarely available. As always, collection of data on fungal infections depends on a number of interested individuals. The problem is particularly acute in the tropics where larger numbers of all forms of fungal infection occur, but there are correspondingly fewer people trained in medical mycology or related subjects. A major feature of fungal disease is therefore under reporting and under diagnosis.

The problems which beset epidemiology in mycology of necessity involve therapy. It is becoming increasingly important to use standardised criteria for pretreatment diagnosis and post-treatment assessment so that the effect of drug therapy can be recorded and valid comparisons made between responses of different patients. Because of the problems of diagnosis, treatment in many cases, and particularly in systemic opportunist infections, has to be instituted before the diagnosis is firmly established because of the risk of leaving a potentially fatal infection untreated. Improvements in this area depend on better methods of diagnosis and agreement on criteria used to assess each infection (Dismukes et al., 1980).

Conclusions

The problems associated with the mycoses are by no means unique or static. At any time difficulties in an area of mycology may be solved, but fresh problems remain in plentiful supply. However throughout the field there is a constant and necessary interplay between diagnosis and management, for treatment cannot properly be instituted without a diagnosis. Many of the problems in medical mycology can be summarised in terms of increasing our ability to diagnose a fungal infection. Our difficulties may be compounded by the need for early diagnosis or the poor state of the patient, but the basic goal remains the diagnosis on which treatment depends.

References

Baker, R.D.: Leukopenia and therapy in leukemia as factors predisposing to fatal mycoses. American Journal of Clinical Pathology 37: 358 (1962).

Burton, J.R.; Zachery, J.B.; Bessin, R.; Rathbun, H.K.; Greenough, W.B.; Sterioff, S.; Wright, J.R.; Slavin, R.E. and Williams, G.M.: Aspergillosis in four renal transplant recipients. Diagnosis and effective treatment with amphotericin B. Annals of Internal Medicine 77: 383 (1972).

Campbell, G.D.: Primary pulmonary cryptococcosis. American Review of Respiratory Disease 94: 236 (1966).

Cantanzaro, A.; Spittle, L. and Moser, K.M.: Immunotherapy of Coccidioidomycosis. Journal of Clinical Investigation 51: 690 (1974).

Cox, R.A.: Immunologic studies in patients with histoplasmosis. American Review of Respiratory Disease 120: 143 (1979).

Cox, R.A. and Arnold, D.R.: Immunoglobulin E in histoplasmosis. Infection and Immunity 29: 290 (1980).

Dismukes, W.E.; Bennett, J.E.; Drutz, D.J.; Graybill, J.R.; Remington, J.S. and Stevens, D.A.: Criteria for evaluation of therapeutic response to antifungal drugs. Reviews of Infectious Diseases 2: 535 (1980).

Drutz, D.J. and Cantanzaro, A.: Coccidioidomycosis Part I. American Review of Respiratory Disease 117: 559 (1978a).

Drutz, D.J. and Cantanzaro, A.: Coccidioidomycosis Part II. American Review of Respiratory Diseases 117: 727 (1978b).

Findlay, G.H. and Vismer, H.F.: Black grain mycetoma. A study of the chemistry, formation and significance of the tissue grain in *Madurella mycetomi* infection. British Journal of Dermatology 91: 297 (1974).

Fishman, L.S.; Griffin, J.R.; Sapico, F.L. and Hecht, R.: Haematogenous Candida endophthalmitis — a complication of candidemia. New England Journal of Medicine 286: 675 (1972).

Furcolow, M.L.: (1957) quoted by Larsh, H.W.: The public health importance of histoplasmosis; in Histoplasmosis. Proceedings of the Second National Conference p.9 (Thomas, Illinois 1971).

Gartenberg, G.; Bottone, E.J.; Keusch, G.T. and Weitzman, I.: Hospital acquired mucormycosis *(Rhizopus rhizopodiformis)* of skin and subcutaneous tissue. New England Journal of Medicine 299: 1115 (1978).

Gentles, J.C. and Holmes, J.G.: Foot ringworm in coal-miners. British Journal of Industrial Medicine 14: 22 (1957).

Goodwin, R.A.; Owens, F.T.; Snell, J.D.; Hubbard, W.W.; Buchanan, D.; Terry, R.T. and des Prez, R.M.: Chronic pulmonary histoplasmosis. Medicine 55: 413 (1976).

Gordon, M.A. and Vedder, D.K.: Serologic tests in diagnosis and prognosis of cryptococcosis. Journal of the American Medical Assocation 197: 961 (1966).

Grin, E.I.: A controlled field trial in Yugoslavia of the efficacy of griseofulvin in the mass treatment of tinea capitis. Bulletin of the World Health Organisation 26: 797 (1962).

Hanifin, J.M.; Ray, L.F. and Lobitz, W.C.: Immunologic reactivity in dermatophytosis. British Journal of Dermatology 90: 1 (1974).

Hay, R.J. and Brostoff, J.: Immune responses in patients with chronic *Trichophyton rubrum* infections. Clinical and Experimental Dermatology 2: 373 (1977).

Hay, R.J.; Mackenzie, D.W.R.; Campbell, C.K. and Philpot, C.M.: Cryptococcosis in the United Kingdom and the Irish Republic: an analysis of 89 cases. Journal of Infection 2: 13 (1980).

Hildick-Smith, G.; Blank, H. and Sarkany, I.: Fungus Diseases and their Treatment, p.31 (Little, Brown, Boston 1964).

Hurley, R. and de Louvois, J.: Candida vaginitis. Postgraduate Medical Journal 55: 645 (1979).

Ichinose, H.: Subcutaneous abscesses due to brown fungi; in Baker (Ed) The Pathologic Anatomy of Mycoses, p.719 (Springer-Verlag, Berlin 1971).

Jennison, R.J.: Thrush in infancy. Archives of Disease in Childhood 52: 747 (1977).

Kauffman, C.A.; Israel, K.S.; Smith, J.W.; White, A.C.; Schwarz, J. and Brooks, G.F.: Histoplasmosis in immunosuppressed patients. American Journal of Medicine 64: 923 (1978).

Kozinn, P.J.; Taschdjian, C.L.; Goldberg, P.K.; Protzmann, W.P.; Mackenzie, D.W.R.; Remington, J.S.; Anderson, S. and Seelig, M.S.: Efficiency of serologic tests in the diagnosis of systemic candidiasis. American Journal of Clinical Pathology 70: 893 (1978).

Krick, J.A. and Remington, J.S.: Opportunistic invasive fungal infections in patients with leukaemia lymphoma. Clinics in Haematology 5: 249 (1976).

Larsh, H.W.; Hall, N.K. and Schlitzer, R.L.: Dynamics of cryptococcal infection by the airborne route. Proceedings of the 4th International Conference on Mycoses (PAHO) Scientific Publication 356: 199 (1978).

Mahgoub, E.S.: Medical management of mycetoma. Bulletin of the World Health Organisation 54: 303 (1976).

Mahgoub, E.S. and Murray, I.G.: Mycetoma, (Heinemann, London 1973).

Mariat, F.: Sur la distribution geographique et la repartition des agents des mycetomes. Bulletin de la Société de Pathologie Exotique 56: 35 (1963).

Masur, H.; Rosen, P.P. and Armstrong, D.: Pulmonary disease caused by Candida species. American Journal of Medicine 63: 914 (1978).

Miller, G.G.; Witwer, M.W.; Braude, A.I. and Davis, C.E.: Rapid identification of *Candida albicans* septicaemia in man by gas-liquid chromatography. Journal of Clinical Investigation 54: 1235 (1974).

Mirsky, H.S. and Cuttner, J.: Fungal infection in acute leukemia. Cancer 30: 348 (1972).

Moore, M.K.: Skin and nail infections caused by non-dermatophyte filamentous fungi. Mykosen (Suppl. I): 128 (1978).

Newberry, W.M.; Walter, J.E.; Chandler, J.W.and Tosh, F.E.: Epidemiologic study of *Cryptococcus neoformans*. Annals of Internal Medicine 67: 724 (1967).

Palmer, C.E.; Edwards, P.Q. and Allfather, W.E.: Characteristics of skin reactions to coccidioidin and histoplasmin with evidence of an unidentified source of sensitisation. American Journal of Hygiene 66: 196 (1957).

Restrepo, A.; Robledo, M.; Ospina, S.; Restrepo, M. and Correa, A.: Distribution of paracoccidioidin sensitivity in Colombia. American Journal of Tropical Medicine and Hygiene 17: 25 (1968).

Rosenbaum, R.B.; Barber, J.V. and Stevens, D.A.: *Candida albicans* pneumonia. Diagnosis by pulmonary aspiration, recovery with treatment. American Review of Respiratory Disease 109: 373 (1974).

Sarosi, G.A.; Hammerman, K.H.; Tosh, F.E. and Kronenberg, P.S.: Clinical features of acute pulmonary blastomycosis. New England Journal of Medicine 290: 540 (1974).

Segal, E.; Berg, R.A.; Pizzo, P.A. and Bennett, J.E.: Detection of Candida antigen in sera of patients with candidiasis by an enzyme-linked immunosorbent assayinhibition technique. Journal of Clinical Microbiology 10: 116 (1979).

Soyinka, F.: Epidemiologic study of dermatophyte infections in Nigeria. Clinical survey and laboratory investigations. Mycopathologia 63: 99 (1979).

Spickard, A.; Butler, W.T.; Andriole, V. and Utz, J.P.: The improved prognosis of cryptococcal meningitis with amphotericin B. Annals of Internal Medicine 58: 66 (1963).

Standard, P.G. and Kaufman, L.: Immunological procedure for the rapid and specific identification of *Coccidioides immitis* cultures. Journal of Clinical Microbiology 5: 149 (1977).

Stobo, J.; Paul, S.; Van Scoy, R.E. and Hermans, P.: Suppressor thymus-derived lymphocytes in fungal infection. Journal of Clinical Investigation 57: 319 (1976).

Chapter II

Current Therapies for Mycotic Diseases

H.E. Jones

Almost 150 years ago Gruby described favus and isolated its aetiological agent, thus introducing mycology as the first of the microbiological sciences. In the years that followed, mycotic infection was recognised as a highly prevalent public health problem. Infected individuals sought aid and the physicians and pharmacists of the day responded with numerous remedies. Most were low potency topical formulations with marginal efficacy. Two of these empirically derived antifungals, potassium iodide — 1903, and Whitfield's Ointment — 1907, have survived the test of time and are still widely used today.

The development of potent antimycotic agents has proceeded much more slowly. Antibiotics inhibit a physiological process which is critical only to the micro-organism and thus selectively inhibit or kill the pathogen without harming the human. Because of the many fundamental differences between the physiology of eukaryotic mammals and the prokaryotic bacteria it has been relatively easy to develop antibacterial agents (table I). These agents are for the most part potent, efficacious, and safe. Fungi, like man, are eukaryotic and both possess similar highly evolved, complex metabolic processes. Whereas the development of antibacterial agents has been relatively easy, the similarities between people and fungi appear to have made the development of antimycotics difficult and slow. In any event, the scientific development of antimycotics has lagged behind the development of antibacterials.

In the past 30 years, certain differences between man and fungi have been exploited for therapeutic advantage. Most of the available antifungals were developed in this period (table II). The first truly potent antimycotics, nystatin and its related polyene, amphotericin B, were developed in the early 1950's. By the late 1950's griseofulvin, the first orally effective antifungal (but with a narrow spectrum of activity), had been introduced to clinical medicine. A decade later the simultaneous, independent development of the first broad spectrum antifungals, miconazole and clotrimazole heralded another major therapeutic advance. However, even these have features which limit their clinical usefulness.

Table I. Some characteristics of fungi, bacteria and man

	Nuclear organisation	Method of reproduction	Cell wall	Major membrane lipid	Cellular nutrition	Lysine metabolism
Bacteria	Prokaryotic	Only mitosis	Present	Hydroxylated glycerols	Mostly absorption	Absorption or diaminopimelate pathway synthesis
Fungi	Eukaryotic	Zygotic meiosis	Present	Ergosterol	More selective absorption	Biosynthesis via α aminoadipic acid pathway
Man	Eukaryotic	Zygotic meiosis	Absent	Cholesterol	Selective absorption and regulated transport to cell	Essential amino acid

This chapter reviews some of the antimycotics available at present and in discussing factors which limit their clinical usefulness focuses attention on the therapeutic problems it is hoped newer compounds, such as ketoconazole, will solve.

Antimycotic Agents in Common Use at Present

Amphotericin B

Amphotericin B from *Streptomyces nodosus* was first isolated in 1955 from the Orinoco River region of Venezuela. It was the second polyene discovered and in many ways it is similar to nystatin and other related tetraenes. Amphotericin B is insoluble in water at neutral pH. The solubility of the deep yellow prisms is increased in sodium desoxycholate, acidic or alkaline conditions, and in dimethylsulphoxide.

Although most fungi are susceptible to low levels of amphotericin B, the degree of sensitivity varies considerably. Fungal susceptibility may relate to the sterol content of the organism's plasma membrane, since the drug acts by binding to a sterol moiety in the cell membrane (p.25). Common fungi sensitive *in vitro* to concentrations of 1µg/ml or less include *Candida* sp., *Blastomyces dermatitidis* and *braziliensis*, *Coccidioides immitis*, *Histoplasma capsulatum*, *Cryptococcus neoformans*, *Torulopsis glabrata*

Table II. Development and clinical spectrum of the various antifungals

Year developed	Generic drug	Type(s) of infection for which drug is principally used[1]				
		superficial[2]	dermatophytosis	candidosis	locally invasive	viscera; and systemic
1903	Potassium iodide				Lymphangetic sporotrichosis	
1907	Whitfield's ointment	±	+			
1940	Undecylenic acid		+			
1949/50	Nystatin			+		
1950	Hydroxystilbamidine					North American blastomycoses
1954/56	8-Hydroxyquinoline derivatives		+	±		
1957	Amphotericin B			+	+	+
1958	Griseofulvin		+			
1958/60	Pimaricin				Mycotic keratitis	
1961	Acrisorcin		+			
1963	Haloprogin		+	±		
1963/68	Tolnaftate		+			
1963/68	Flucytosine			+	± *Cladiosporium* sp.	Cryptococcosis
1969/70	Miconazole	+	+	+	+	+
1969/70	Clotrimazole	+	+	+		
1974/75	Econazole	+	+	+		

1   + = general effectiveness   ± = limited effectiveness.
2   Includes pityriasis versicolor and tinea nigra palmaris.

and *Sporotrichum schenkii*. The sensitivity of *Aspergillus* strains is variable. Resistance of *Candida* to amphotericin B can be induced *in vitro*, but there is no evidence that resistance occurs *in vivo*.

Amphotericin B is poorly absorbed from the gastrointestinal tract, and requires slow intravenous administration. Some other pharmacokinetic properties of the drug are summarised in table III.

Toxicity is a frequent problem with amphotericin B (Maddux and Barriere, 1980). Some degree of azotaemia almost always occurs with intravenous administration, and may be dose-limiting. Although renal function returns toward normal on discontinuing therapy, some residual impairment may occur; the degree of renal damage may be related to the total dose of the drug administered. Hypokalaemia also occurs frequently, and may become symptomatic if uncorrected. Decreased haematocrit occurs in almost all patients during therapy, but the normochromic, normocytic anaemia produced is self-limiting. Leukopenia, thrombocytopenia and allergic reactions occur rarely.

Despite its toxicity, the necessity of careful monitoring of renal function and serum potassium, and the inconvenience of intravenous administration which may be accompanied by thrombophlebitis, amphotericin B has been the treatment of choice for many locally invasive and systemic infections.

Flucytosine

Flucytosine, a fluorinated pyrimidine, is a white crystalline material slightly to moderately soluble in water. Its range of antifungal activity is limited: *Candida albicans, Cryptococcus neoformans, Torulopsis glabrata,* and some *Cladosporium* and Phialophora species are usually sensitive to it (Bennett, 1977), although naturally resistant strains are found among these species. Unfortunately, in most fungal infections (excepting chromomycosis) flucytosine-resistant strains may emerge rapidly if the drug is used alone, thus limiting its usefulness (Block et al., 1973). It is used primarily in combination with amphotericin B, especially in cryptococcal meningitis (Bennett et al., 1979).

Flucytosine is better absorbed from the gut than might be predicted from its moderate solubility in water (Polak, 1979), and the drug is marketed only in an oral dose form. It reaches the cerebrospinal fluid in relatively high concentrations (table III). Flucytosine is excreted almost entirely in unchanged form in the urine, and dosage must be adjusted accordingly in patients with renal dysfunction; in anuria the elimination half-life is variably extended to 28 to 430 hours, compared with 3 to 8 hours in normal renal function (Heel and Avery, 1980b).

Side effects are not common, and when they do occur are usually mild. Occasionally, however, serious toxicity occurs, such as bowel perforation; leukopenia and thrombocytopenia have been reported. Haematological abnormalities seem to be related to serum concentrations of the drug in excess of $100\mu g/ml$ (see Medoff and Kobayashi, 1980); blood level monitoring is probably advisable, especially in patients with renal dysfunction.

Griseofulvin

Griseofulvin is an antifungal antibiotic produced by *Penicillium griseofulvum*. Although first isolated in the 1930's and used to some extent as an agricultural fungicide, it was not until 20 years later that griseofulvin was introduced to medicine, becoming the first potent oral antifungal. The crystals are practically insoluble in water and only slightly soluble in ethanol.

Griseofulvin's fungistatic activity is limited to actively growing dermatophytes. For many years griseofulvin has been the standard therapy for all forms of human and animal dermatophytosis which cannot be cleared with topical therapy.

Microbial resistance has been associated with griseofulvin treatment (Fisher et al., 1961) and natural resistance of certain strains is recognised (Hildick-Smith et al., 1964). The prevalence and clinical significance of resistance to griseofulvin and whether it is caused by induction or selection has not been defined (Artis et al., 1981).

Griseofulvin is not effective topically, even though topical application in an organic solvent provides excellent penetration to the site of the infection (Munro, 1967). This is an enigma for when given orally, the active agent must gain access to the same site in order to inhibit the organism. After oral dosing, griseofulvin is delivered to the stratum corneum via the sweat or by deposition in keratinocytes. It is tempting to speculate that a metabolite of the orally administered drug may be the active agent within the skin.

Table III. Summary of pharmacokinetic properties of some systemic antifungal drugs (after Heel and Avery, 1980a)

Drug	Oral bioavailability	Elimination half-life (hours)	Apparent volume of distribution (L/kg)	Protein binding (%)	CSF penetration	Elimination pattern
Amphotericin B	Low	24-48[1]	~4	> 90	Low	Urinary excretion of inactivated drug[2]
Clotrimazole	Low[3]	~4		~98		
Flucytosine	High	3-8	~0.7	2-4	High[4]	Urinary excretion of unchanged drug
Griseofulvin	Variable[5]	10-24	1-2			Primarily urinary excretion of metabolites
Miconazole	Low	~24	~21	~98	Low[6]	

1 A much longer half-life (~360 hours) can be calculated if slow release from tissues is allowed for.
2 Details of metabolic pathways are not known.
3 Extensive hepatic clearance of absorbed drug — see text.
4 CSF levels are about 70 to 80% of simultaneous plasma levels (Polak, 1979).
5 Highly dependent on particle size of the dosage form used (Lin and Symchowicz, 1975) — see text.
6 Variable values reported of about 3 to 48% of serum concentrations (Heel et al., 1980).

Confusion has arisen over oral absorption and dosage (see table III). The original 500mg tablets were considered approximately equal to 250mg of micronised griseofulvin and to 125mg of the ultramicronised form, but many clinicians question the clinical equivalence of these doses.

Adverse effects are frequent but rarely serious. Hepatomas have been produced in mice but not in other species. In man, headache, which can be severe, occurs most frequently; gastrointestinal disturbances and photosensitivity occur occasionally. The more serious problems are rare, and include porphyria, oestrogen-like effects, leukopenia, aggravation of lupus erythematosus, and interference with concomitantly administered warfarin-like anticoagulants.

Hydroxystilbamidine

Hydroxystilbamidine isethionate, is a yellow crystalline material which is freely soluble in water. It is active again *Blastomyces dermatitidis* both *in vivo* and *in vitro*. It has little activity against most other pathogenic fungi although it is active against some protozoa, e.g. *Leishmania* species. The drug is administered intravenously over several weeks until a total dose of 8g has been given. Adverse effects are common and include malaise, anorexia, nausea, and headache, as well as more serious hepatic toxicity (see Utz, 1980). More potent and safer antifungals will replace this drug if they have not done so already.

Imidazole Antifungals

The imidazole group of antifungal agents are of considerable importance in clinical practice. Their broad spectrum of antifungal activity, covering most pathogenic fungi (for review see Heel et al., 1978, 1980; Sawyer et al., 1975a,b), has provided an important advance in antifungal therapy. They also have some activity against Gram-positive bacteria.

Clotrimazole

Clotrimazole is a substituted imidazole which is only slightly soluble in water but soluble in common organic solvents. Clotrimazole is absorbed from the gastrointestinal tract to some degree as one might predict from its solubility pattern. Interestingly and disappointingly, the drug when given orally induces hepatic microsomal enzymes, notably cytochrome P_{450}, with a subsequent decrease in serum levels of the drug. After a few days of oral dosing no drug can be detected in the serum. Used chiefly as a 1% cream or lotion for topical use, its efficacy and adverse effects are comparable to those of miconazole (see below).

Econazole

Econazole, an imidazole derivative which like clotrimazole is essentially used only topically, is effective in a wide variety of superficial fungal infections (Heel et al., 1978). It has been administered systemically to a small number of patients with deep mycoses with mixed results, but its systemic use was superseded by the development of a parenteral formulation of miconazole (see below). In vaginal candidosis econazole has been used both in a 'traditional' 2-week treatment course, and in a short term higher dose course given over 3 days (Balmer, 1976), with comparable results. The shorter course partially (but not completely) alleviates the inconvenience of topical therapy for a vaginal infection. Econazole is well tolerated on local application, with only occasional reports of reactions such as irritation, burning or itching.

Miconazole

Miconazole, a substituted imidazole only slightly soluble in water, and its distant cousin, clotrimazole, were the first truly broad spectrum antifungals. Practically all pathogenic yeast and fungi are sensitive *in vitro* to low levels of miconazole. The drug is available for topical use as miconazole nitrate and for intravenous use as miconazole base dissolved in polyethoxylated castor oil and water. The parenteral use of miconazole represents a real advance in the treatment of extensive cutaneous, invasive and systemic mycoses (Heel et al., 1980). Miconazole is only partially absorbed after oral administration, with oral bioavailability of about 25 to 30% (Bolaert et al., 1976). It reaches many body fluids in significant concentrations, but unfortunately cerebrospinal fluid concentrations are low. As with econazole and clotrimazole, side effects from topical therapy are minimal, but parenteral therapy produces several problems. Phlebitis has occurred frequently in some studies, and may be related to the formulation of the drug. Nausea, fever and chills, rash and pruritus also occur. Pruritus may be particularly severe and persistent in some patients. Haematological abnormalities, which in some cases were possibly related to the polyethoxylated castor oil carrier solution, have been reported in a number of patients (Stevens et al., 1976; Stevens, 1977). Hyponatraemia, giving rise to severe symptoms in a few cases, has also occurred especially in patients with meningitis (Stevens, 1977).

Nystatin

Nystatin was the first polyene antibiotic and the first truly potent anticandidal antifungal. Nystatin and cyclohexidine were both isolated from *Streptomyces noursei*. Nystatin is a light yellow powder which is completely insoluble in water.

Although most fungal pathogens are inhibited *in vitro* by low concentrations of nystatin, its insolubility and systemic toxicity have restricted its use primarily to topical and mucosal *Candida* infections. When administered orally, there is no absorption; hence, only the gastrointestinal tract and its contents are subject to its antimycotic effects.

Pimaricin

Pimaricin is a polyene which is related to nystatin and amphotericin B. This tetraene is extracted from *Streptomyces natalensis*. Pimaricin is a colourless crystalline material which is insoluble in water and the common organic solvents. It is active against a variety of fungi including many which produce ocular infections, especially keratitis. Since few antifungal agents inhibit these corneal pathogens, pimaricin plays a unique role in the therapy of mycotic keratitis.

Potassium Iodide

In 1903, de Beurmann and Gougerot wrote of the effectiveness of potassium iodide in the treatment of sporotrichosis. Today it is still the treatment of choice for the cutaneous, lymphangetic form of sporotrichosis. However, it is usually ineffective in other clinical forms of sporotrichosis, and other fungal infections do not respond to iodide therapy. Potassium iodide is usually administered as drops of a saturated solution of potassium iodide.

When its antifungal effect was first appreciated, potassium iodide was already known to promote resolution of granulomatous lesions caused by syphilis and tuberculosis. It may be that it exerts its beneficial effect on the host-parasite struggle by action on host tissues or processes. Intracellular killing may be dependent on oxidative processes which appear to require iodine. Alternatively, iodine may act on the complement cascade to facilitate neutrophil chemotaxis to the site of infection.

Side effects of therapy are generally mild and include acneform eruptions, parotiditis, and gastrointestinal intolerance. Iodism can occur frequently, but is usually responsive to a brief interruption in therapy or a reduced dose.

Tolnaftate

Tolnaftate is a crystalline compound which is insoluble in water. *In vitro* it shows potent activity against dermatophytes but is without activity against yeasts or other pathogens. Tolnaftate is marketed as a topical agent for dermatophytosis. Its clinical effectiveness is less than its *in vitro* activity would lead one to predict.

Whitfield's Ointment

By 1907 when his handbook of skin diseases and treatments was published, Arthur Whitfield had already established the efficacy of his antifungal ointment. The ointment, a mixture of 12% benzoic acid and 6% salicylic acid, may act directly on dermatophytes or promote desquamation and healing by its keratolytic effect. Interestingly, both salicylic and benzoic acids are, in keeping with their fellow antifungals, only slightly soluble in water. Today, its main advantage is its low cost, for there are more potent antifungals available. Also, Whitfield's Ointment may cause irritation and if applied over large areas, systemic absorption of salicylic acid may lead to toxicity.

The Problem of Drug Insolubility

Many antifungals including most of those discussed in this chapter share the property of being almost insoluble in water (table IV). Only acrisorcin (not discussed in the text since it is not widely used), hydroxystilbamidine, and potassium iodide can be classified as soluble with the latter two agents being freely soluble in water. Interestingly, these three agents have little in common except that they are not highly efficacious.

Perhaps there is a message in the fact that most antifungals are insoluble in water but soluble in some organic solvents. Solubility in organic solvents often mirrors lipid solubility which may facilitate drug interaction with the lipid-rich fungal membranes. In any event, poor solubility in water and body fluids renders these drugs difficult to work with and limits their potential dose forms (table IV). Poor solubility may also retard absorption and limit blood levels.

Alternatively, lipid affinity may enhance toxicity by damaging host membranes. For some antifungals, particularly the polyenes, this may explain much of their toxicity.

The three antifungals with limited solubility in water, namely, griseofulvin, flucytosine, and clotrimazole are each absorbed well enough to permit use in an oral dose form.

Of the practically insoluble agents (table IV), only amphotericin B and miconazole have been successfully formulated into either an aqueous suspension or special vehicle for parenteral use. The remaining anti-fungals in the table are marketed in a topical dose form only. The large amount of sebaceous and epidermal lipids present in the skin may facilitate cutaneous penetration of these lipophilic, hydrophobic substances.

Factors Which Limit the Clinical Usefulness of the Various Antifungals

In retrospect, it is easy to see that the major problem with 19th century antifungal remedies was their marginal efficacy. It is more difficult to assess the relative efficacy and problems of the more recently developed antifungals. This is true in large part because analysis of the published data is hampered by the fact that *in vitro* test systems are not standardised. The medium used, conditions of incubation, the solvent for the antifungal, and even the test organisms vary from laboratory to laboratory.

It is even more difficult to compare clinical trials. Different doses, dosage schedules, infection syndromes, fungal strains, the ever present human factor, and the patient's occupation and environment make accurate comparison of results impossible.

Nevertheless, it is clear that when used appropriately for suitable indications amphotericin B, griseofulvin, the imidazoles and nystatin are potent *in vitro* and clinically efficacious. Even these agents are not without problems that limit their usefulness, some of which are discussed in detail below.

The antifungal spectrum of griseofulvin limits its use to the dermatophytes although there are some forms of dermatophytosis which respond poorly to the recommended doses. Failure to resolve *Trichophyton rubrum* infection has recently been correlated with *in vitro* microbial resis-

Table IV. The relationship between solubility of an antifungal and its marketed formulation(s)

Solubility in water	Topical dose forms	Intravenous dose forms	Oral dose forms
Soluble	Acrisorcin	Hydroxystilbamidine	Potassium iodide
Limited solubility	Clotrimazole		Flucytosine Griseofulvin
Practically insoluble	Pimaricin, Nystatin, Miconazole, Econazole, Amphotericin B, Hydroxyquinoline, Whitfield's ointment, Undecyclenic acid, Tolnaftate, Haloprogin	Miconazole Amphotericin B	

Table V. Factors which may limit the usefulness of the available antifungals

1. Low potency
2. Poor solubility in water or body fluids
3. Limited, inconvenient dose forms
4. Narrow clinical spectrum
5. Emergence of microbial resistance
6. Toxicity or poor patient tolerance

tance to griseofulvin (Artis et al., 1981). The adverse effects of griseofulvin, although mainly only a nuisance, may preclude or interrupt therapy.

Amphotericin B is the standard therapy and in the past has often been the only treatment for many serious, life-threatening fungal infections, e.g. coccidioidomycosis, histoplasmosis, etc. The intravenous dose form requires hospitalisation which greatly increases the cost of therapy. Amphotericin B also has predictable adverse effects which may preclude and often interrupt therapy. Numerous side effects occur including serious toxicity and even death. As a topical agent, amphotericin B is of little value in the treatment of candidosis and the drug is not active against the dermatophytes.

Of the available imidazoles, miconazole is the most useful drug for systemic infections. Enzyme induction and toxicity when administered intravenously limits the use of clotrimazole to the topical route. In the topical dose form, miconazole and clotrimazole are of approximately equal efficacy. Parenteral miconazole is effective against several locally invasive and systemic mycoses, although its relative efficacy compared with amphotericin B has not been well established. Enzyme induction is not a significant clinical problem with miconazole, but adverse effects from parenteral miconazole are not uncommon and frequently interrupt therapy.

Thus, one or more of the factors in table V affect all of the antifungals in use at present.

Because of these problems, there are types of fungal infection which respond poorly or cannot be successfully and safely treated. Some locally invasive infections, several systemic mycoses and even some forms of dermatomycosis are not eradicated by conventional drug therapy. This may be the case even though no adverse effects hamper or constrain therapy. As an obvious example, chronic, widespread tinea corporis and erythrodermic tinea pedis are frequently recalcitrant. Topical application is difficult in extensive infection but therapeutic failure may occur even when compliance is assured by having medical personnel apply the most effective topical medicaments. Even high dose oral griseofulvin combined with topical imidazoles fails to resolve some subtypes of dermatophytosis.

Patients with chronic, stabilised fungal infections resistant to therapy are usually found to have compromised or defective host resistance. This is true for the superficial infections as well as the systemic mycoses. Even with clinical and mycological resolution of an adequately treated infection, relapse and/or reinfection is the rule. The cost of treating recalcitrant fungal infection is high; for many patients it is prohibitive. Highly efficacious, more easily administered and less toxic antifungals would be welcomed by physicians and patients who must contend with life-threatening infections or those infections which drastically reduce the quality of life.

References

Artis, W.M.; Odle, B.M. and Jones, H.E.: Griseofulvin-resistant dermatophytosis correlates with *in vitro* resistance. Archives of Dermatology 117: 16-19 (1981).

Balmer, J.A.: Three-day therapy of vulvovaginal candidosis with econazole: a multicentric study comprising 996 cases. American Journal of Obstetrics and Gynecology 126: 436 (1976).

Bennett, J.E.: Drugs five years later: Flucytosine. Annals of Internal Medicine 86: 319 (1977).

Bennett, J.E.; Dismukes, W.E.; Duma, R.J. et al.: Amphotericin B-flucytosine in cryptococcal meningitis. New England Journal of Medicine 301: 126 (1979).

Block, E.R.; Jennings, A.E. and Bennett, J.E.: 5-Fluorocytosine resistance in *Cryptococcus neoformans*. Antimicrobial Agents and Chemotherapy 3: 649-656 (1973).

Bolaert, J.; Daneels, R.; Van Landuyt, H. and Symoens, J.: Miconazole plasma levels in healthy subjects and in patients with impaired renal function. Chemotherapy 6: 165 (1976).

Fisher, B.K.; Smith, J.G.; Crounse, R.G. et al.: Verrucous epidermophytosis: Its response and resistance to griseofulvin. Archives of Dermatology 84: 375-380 (1961).

Heel, R.C.; Brogden, R.N.; Speight, T.M. and Avery, G.S.: Econazole: a review of its antifungal activity and therapeutic efficacy. Drugs 16: 117-201 (1978).

Heel, R.C. and Avery, G.S.: Appendix A. Drug data information; in Avery (Ed) Drug Treatment, 2nd Edition, pp.1211-1222 (Adis Press, Sydney; Churchill Livingstone, Edinburgh 1980a).

Heel, R.C. and Avery, G.S.: Appendix E. Guide to drug dosage in renal failure; in Avery (Ed) Drug Treatment, 2nd Edition, pp.1290-1303 (Adis Press, Sydney; Churchill-Livingstone, Edinburgh 1980b).

Heel, R.C.; Brogden, R.N.; Pakes, G.E.; Speight, T.M. and Avery, G.S.: Miconazole: a preliminary review of its therapeutic efficacy in systemic fungal infections. Drugs 19: 7-30 (1980).

Hildick-Smith, G.; Blank, H. and Sarkany, I.: Fungus Diseases and Their Treatment (Churchill, London 1964).

Lin, C. and Symchowicz, S.: Absorption, distribution, metabolism and excretion of griseofulvin in man and animals. Drug Metabolism Reviews 4: 75 (1975).

Maddux, M.S. and Barriere, S.L.: A review of complications of amphotericin-B therapy: Recommendations for prevention and management. Drug Intelligence and Clinical Pharmacy 14: 177 (1980).

Medoff, G. and Kobayashi, G.S.: Strategies in the management of systemic fungal infections. New England Journal of Medicine 302: 145-155 (1980).

Munro, D.D. and Stoughton, R.B.: Dimethylacetamide (DMAC) and dimethylformamide (DMFA) effect on percutaneous absorption. Archives of Dermatology 92: 585 (1965).

Polak, A.: Pharmacokinetics of amphotericin B and flucytosine. Postgraduate Medical Journal 55: 667 (1979).

Sawyer, P.R.: Brogden, R.N.; Pinder, R.M.; Speight, T.M. and Avery, G.S.: Miconazole: a review of its antifungal activity and therapeutic efficacy. Drugs 9: 406-423 (1975a).

Sawyer, P.R.; Brogden, R.N.; Pinder, R.M.; Speight, T.M. and Avery, G.S.: Clotrimazole: a review of its antifungal activity and therapeutic efficacy. Drugs 9: 424-447 (1975b).

Schar, G.; Kayser, F.H. and Dupont, M.C.: Antimicrobial activity of econazole and miconazole *in vitro* and in experimental candidiasis and aspergillosis. Chemotherapy 22: 211 (1976).

Stevens, D.A.: Miconazole in the treatment of systemic fungal infections. American Review of Respiratory Disease 116: 801 (1977).

Stevens, D.A.; Levine, M.B. and Deresinski, S.C.: Miconazole in coccidioidomycosis: II. Therapeutic and pharmacologic studies in man. American Journal of Medicine 60: 191 (1976).

Thienpont, D.; van Cutsem, J.; van Nueten, J.M.; Niemegeers, C.J.E. and Marsboom, R.: Biological and toxicological properties of econazole, a broad-spectrum antimycotic. Arzneimittel-Forschung 25: 224 (1975).

Utz, J.P.: Chemotherapy for the systemic mycoses: the prelude to ketoconazole. Reviews of Infectious Diseases 2: 625-632 (1980).

Chapter III

The Mode of Action of Antifungal Drugs

M. Borgers and
H. Van den Bossche

Over the last few years a substantial number of papers has been published in which the mode of action of individual or groups of antifungal drugs has been reviewed (D'Arcy and Scott, 1978; Raab, 1980; Odds, 1979; Heeres and Van den Bossche, 1980). This account of the mode of action will therefore deal briefly with the essential of the above cited literature and focus mainly on recent advances in the field of biochemistry and morphology. The subcellular target or site(s) of drug action is fairly well established for most compounds. The main classes of antifungals used today, comprising the polyene antibiotics, griseofulvin, tolnaftate and the azole derivatives vary greatly from each other as far as their spectrum of activity, potency and safety margin is concerned. These properties are largely determined by their particular mode of action. Depending on the nature and the function of the attained target a drug exerts fungicidal effects or will be merely fungistatic and acts preferentially or uniquely against certain species. The synergistic action between drug and host defence cells and the possible immunomodulating properties which have been recently reported for polyenes and azole derivatives, is of considerable interest, especially in the treatment of deep mycoses (p.29). Other important determinants unrelated to its mode of action that govern the usefulness of an antifungal compound, are its bioavailability and pharmacokinetics after various routes of administration. In this respect ketoconazole, the antifungal profile of which relies basically on the same mechanism of action as the other members of the azole series, is distinguished from the others mainly by its high efficacy after oral administration.

Polyenes

A common chemical characteristic of all polyene antibiotics is a macrolide with a β-hydroxylated portion and a conjugated double bond system in the lactone ring (Lampen, 1966). These polyenes are produced mainly by Streptomycetaceae. Nystatin, amphotericin B, candicidin, pimaricin, trichomycin and hamycin are the best known members of this group (Odds, 1979). The mechanism of action of all the polyenes is essentially the same (Hamilton-Miller, 1973). According to a recent study involving 14 polyene antibiotics and 6 of their derivatives there is a clear correlation between the type of biological action and the size of the polyene macrolide ring. The heptanes cause cell damage resulting in considerable potassium leakage or a fungistatic effect at lower concentrations, whereas higher concentrations provoke cell death. A triene, tetraenes, pentaenes and one hexaene cause little or no potassium leakage or fungistatic effect separable from cell death (Kotler-Brajtburg et al., 1979). Polyenes promote leakage of cellular constituents, an effect that depends on the irreversible binding of the drugs to membrane sterols. The resulting destruction of the membrane integrity impairs uptake mechanisms, induces the loss of potassium, sugars, ammonium, phosphate, carboxylic acids, phosphorus esters, nucleotides and proteins and promotes intracellular acidification (Lampen, 1966). Exposure of *Candida albicans* cultures to amphotericin B disrupts subcellular membrane entities without an obvious disturbance of the cell wall (Borgers, 1980). Differences in susceptibility of various fungi to polyenes have been attributed to a different sterol content of the cell membranes or to variations in cell wall permeability of the drugs. Resistance to polyenes, which has been reported only occasionally, is usually associated with an increase of membrane sterols, in particular ergosterol (Hamilton-Miller, 1972; Woods et al., 1974). The difference in toxicity to fungal and host cells has also been ascribed to the difference in membrane sterols. Polyenes have a somewhat higher affinity for ergosterol, the main sterol of fungal membranes, than for the mammalian cholesterol, hence the relatively selective toxicity (Kitajima et al., 1976).

In addition to its antifungal properties, amphotericin B appears to have immunoadjuvant effects. Experimentally, this polyene enhances the number of antibody-producing cells in the spleen and lymph nodes of mice (Little et al., 1978) and augments delayed hypersensitivity reactions and cell-mediated immunity (Shirley and Little, 1979a,b).

Griseofulvin

Griseofulvin, the antibiotic, isolated from *Penicillium griseofulvum* (Oxford et al., 1939), shows a remarkable fungistatic activity against dermatophytes. Over the years, a variety of effects at different subcellular sites have been proposed to account for its antifungal activity. These include inhibition of the synthesis of hyphal cell wall material (Bent and Moore, 1966; Evans and White, 1967) binding to RNA (Bent and Moore, 1966); interference with nucleic acid synthesis and mitosis (Bent and Moore, 1966; Malawista et al., 1968; Weber et al., 1976) and inhibition of microtubules (Norberg, 1970; Malawista, 1975). In view of the fact that griseofulvin is only active on growing cells the latter hypothesis on the primary interactions with microtubules is very attractive for it may explain some of the previously formulated proposals, i.e. as a blocker of mitosis (spindle microtubules) or lack of adequate renewal of cell wall material (cytoplasmic microtubules). Indeed, there is evidence that griseofulvin not only acts as a spindle poison but also interferes with cytoplasmic microtubules (Malawista, 1975). Considering the role of microtubules in the cytoplasmic transport of secretory material towards the cell periphery (Borgers et al., 1975), one might easily imagine that following their destruction the processing of newly synthetised cell wall constituents at the growing hyphal tips is impaired. The resistance to griseofulvin of fungal species such as *Candida, Cryptococcus, Phialophora* and *Histoplasma* may be due to either absorption by these fungi, to a different sensitivity of their microtubles or a different dependency on an intact microtubular system. There is no reported occurrence of developing resistance of originally sensitive species to griseofulvin (p.17).

Tolnaftate

Tolnaftate is a synthetic drug (Nogushi et al., 1962) in use for the topcial treatment of dermatophytoses. Like griseofulvin, tolnaftate is not active against *Candida* species. The activity of this drug also is demonstrated only in growing cells (Weinstein et al., 1964; Robinson and Raskin, 1965). The mode of action of tolnaftate has not been reported. In view of its similarity to griseofulvin as far as spectrum of activity is concerned, it would be worthwhile determining whether or not this drug interferes with microtubules.

Flucytosine

Flucytosine (5-fluorocytosine), a fluorinated pyrimidine, is the only antifungal in clinical use which is a true antimetabolite. Its activity appears to be limited to yeast-like fungi (*Candida* and *Cryptococcus* species) and to *Aspergillus* (Shadomy, 1969; D'Arcy and Scott, 1978). Flucytosine owes its antifungal property to the fact that the fungal enzymes are to some extent unable to distinguish between fluorinated pyrimidine and their natural analogues. Its mode of action has been thoroughly investigated by Polak and colleagues (Polak and Grenson, 1973a,b; Polak and Scholer 1973a,b, 1975). The drug enters the cell cytoplasm through the action of cytosine permease and becomes deaminated to 5-fluorouracyl by means of cytosine deaminase. The drug's spectrum of activity appears essentially determined by the presence and efficiency of the latter enzyme (Polak and Scholer, 1980). Its low toxicity to the mammalian host is also explained by the lack of cytosine deaminase. 5-Fluorouracyl is then phosphorylated and incorporated into RNA. Another pathway for 5-fluorouracyl emerged from recent investigations and involves the formation of 5-fluorodeoxy-uridine monophosphate which inhibits thymidylate synthetase thereby impairing the biosynthesis of fungal DNA (Polak and Scholer, 1980). So far, no definite conclusion can be drawn from these experiments as to whether the impaired DNA synthesis and the resulting defective cell division or the dysfunction of fungal RNA leading to disturbed protein synthesis are the primary cause of the drug's antifungal activity. Flucytosine's activity against yeasts is antagonised by purine and pyrimidine bases (Polak and Grenson, 1973b; Holt and Newman, 1973; Polak and Scholer, 1975). Resistance to the drug can reportedly be attributed to many factors. Resistant mutants may have either deficient enzyme systems involved with the metabolic pathways of the drug, increased synthesis of competing pyrimidines or compensating mechanisms for the abnormal RNA function (Odds, 1979). The frequency of resistance is furthermore exacerbated by the development of resistance during drug therapy (Warner et al., 1971; Cartwright et al., 1972; Holt and Newman, 1973; Hoeprich et al., 1974). Reports on the ultrastructural modification in fungi and flucytosine are scanty and concern slight folding of the surface of yeast cells (Ansehn et al., 1974) and swelling of the nucleus with the intranuclear appearance of fine filamentous particles (Arai et al., 1977).

Azole Derivatives

Introduced some 12 years ago, the earliest members of the imidazole series, miconazole and clotrimazole (Godefroi et al., 1969; Plempel et al., 1969) have now developed into first choice drugs in the treatment of many mycotic diseases. More recently marketed imidazoles are econazole and isoconazole, which share most of the antifungal properties of their analogue miconazole (Godefroi et al., 1969). Several new imidazole derivatives such as ketoconazole (Heeres et al., 1979; Thienpont et al., 1979) parconazole, tioconazole, sulconazole and butoconazole are at present under investigation (Heeres and Van den Bossche, 1980). Amongst these ketoconazole has been studied extensively by clinicians because of its antifungal efficacy after oral treatment (Levine and Cobb, 1978; Borelli et al., 1979; Symoens et al., 1980). Terconazole is a recently synthesised triazole derivative (Heeres et al., unpublished), with a high fungicidal activity after topical application (Van Cutsem et al., 1980).

The azole derivatives differ from the other antimycotics in their broad spectrum of activity. They are active against dermatophytes, multiphasic fungi and yeasts and are also active against some bacteria and protozoa (Janssen and Van Bever, 1979; Van den Bossche et al., 1980). As far as their mechanism of action is concerned miconazole, clotrimazole and ketoconazole are the most extensively studied azole derivatives, both biochemically and morphologically.

Morphological Changes in Imidazole Treated Microorganisms

Candidosis: The mode of action of various azole derivatives has been primarily investigated using *C. albicans* yeast phase cultures (Iwata et al., 1973; De Nollin and Borgers, 1974, 1975, 1976; Preusser, 1976). Transmission and scanning electron microscopy revealed that after ex-

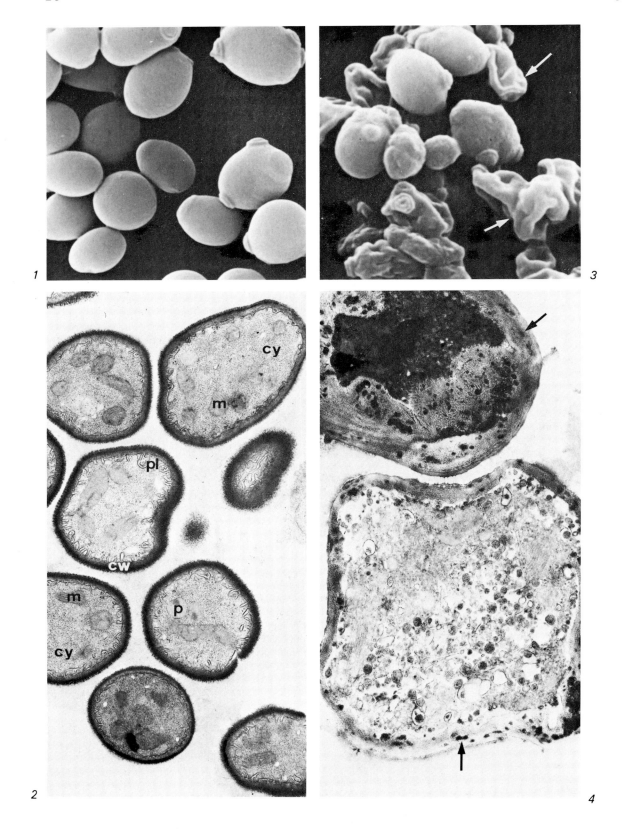

posure to low doses of imidazoles (10-100ng/ml) peculiar changes took place at the plasma membrane and the cell wall. These were unique for this series of compounds. The alterations consisted of the formation of highly osmiophilic vesicles, most probably representing altered membrane constituents, deposited in the cell wall and in the central vacuole. At the same time a large increase in cell volume took place and abnormalities of cell division occurred. The otherwise smooth surface became wrinkled and showed randomly distributed bud scars. The enlarged cells did not separate after normal budding and division. Exposure to higher doses (0.5-50µg/ml) induced deterioration of all subcellular organelles and because of the loss of osmotic resistance the cells became angular in appearance (figs. 1-4). Complete necrosis was induced with 50µg/ml except for the clotrimazole cultures (De Nollin and Borgers, 1976) which were still viable. Fatty overload was one of the characteristic features seen with the high dose regimen.

When *C. albicans* was cultured in its mycelial form (for some strains pseudo-mycelium) [figs. 5 and 6] the effect of the drug on the structural changes was different. The medium used to promote the outgrowth of mycelium from inoculated yeast cells was Eagle's minimum essential medium (EMEM) supplemented with non-essential amino acids and 10% fetal calf serum. Long lasting hyphal growth was obtained when cultures were grown in a humidified atmosphere of 5% CO_2 at 36°C (Borgers et al. 1979a; Aerts et al., 1980). The azole derivatives inhibited this transformation in concentrations ranging between 0.005 and 0.5µg/ml. These low doses, however, permitted a limited outgrowth of clustered yeast cells, but similar membranous changes occurred (fig. 6) as did in the exposed yeast cell cultures (*vide supra*). Higher concentrations of miconazole and ketoconazole (50µg/ml) caused massive necrosis of the inoculated cells, again with fatty overload (figs. 5 and 6). These morphological data suggest that the primary site of action of these drugs is the plasma membrane with the simultaneous involvement of the central vacuolar system. In the higher dose range, the internal organelle disorganisation leading to cell death was interpreted as the consequence of drug induced changes of oxidative and peroxidative enzyme activities resulting in an intracellular build-up of toxic hydrogen peroxide concentrations (Borgers et al., 1977; De Nollin et al., 1977).

Recent experiments with mixed cultures of *C. albicans* and leucocytes revealed a synergistic action between host defence cells and imidazole antifungals (De Brabander et al., 1980). The EMEM used to culture *C. albicans* mycelial phase cells is a medium originally employed for culturing mammalian cells and lends itself extremely well to mixed culture experiments thereby mimicking to some degree a host-pathogen situation. In such a system, polymorphonuclear leucocytes (PMN) and macrophages avidly engulf the yeast phase cells. However, they are unable to eradicate

C. albicans **cultured in a yeast phase supporting medium**

Fig. 1. Control culture. Round and oval shaped cells of equal size are all smooth surfaced. SEM (× 4.000).

Fig. 2. Control culture. Sectioned yeast cells presenting the detailed ultrastructure of the various subcellular organelles such as cell wall (cw), plasmalemma (pl), mitochondria (m), peroxisomes (p), cytosol filled with ribosomes (cy). TEM (× 2.000).

Fig. 3. Culture treated with 10⁻⁴M miconazole. The rough surfaced yeast cells are present in clusters, many of them collapsed (arrows). SEM (× 5.700).

Fig. 4. Culture treated with 10⁻⁵M miconazole. The angular cells are fully necrotised. The degenerated organelles are barely identifiable. Typical phospholipid-like vesicles (arrows) are present in the altered cell wall. TEM (× 16.500).

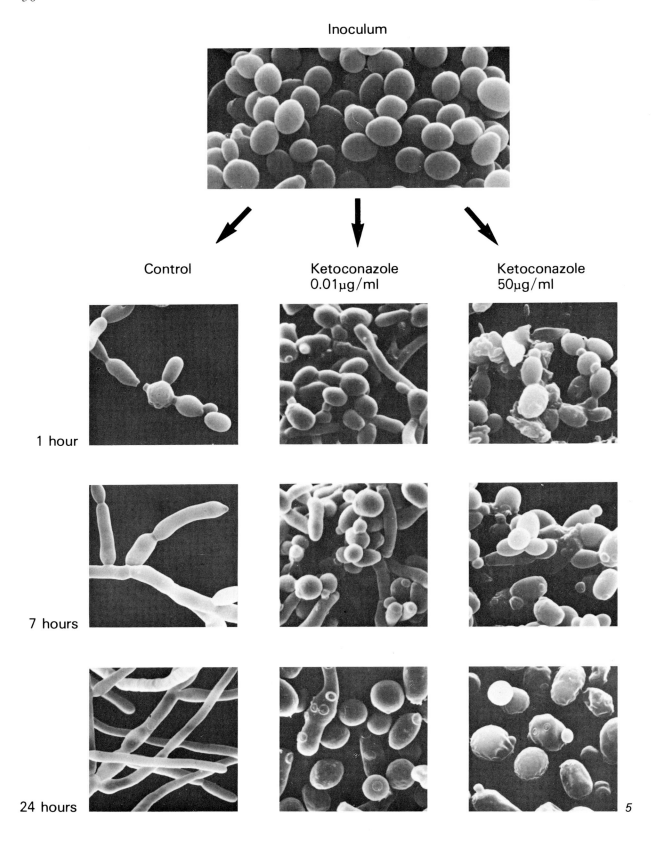

Growth 24 hours

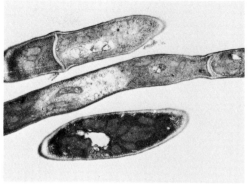

Control

Inoculum

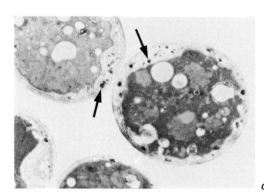

Ketoconazole 0.01µg/ml

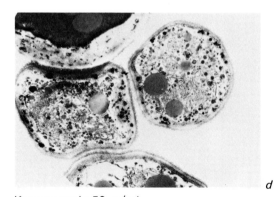

Ketoconazole 50µg/ml

6
_____

Fig. 5. *C. albicans* cultured in a mycelium supporting medium. The time-related development of mycelium from the inoculated yeast cells and the influence of low (0.01µg/ml) and high dose (50µg/ml) ketoconazole on their morphogenetic transformation is shown. SEM (× 2.100).

Fig. 6. Transmission electron micrography of *C. albicans*, cultured as in figure 5. Note that the exposure to a low dose of ketoconazole results in the characteristic deposition of osmiophilic vesicles (arrows) in the cell wall of growth inhibited yeasts whereas a high dose induces complete necrosis of the inoculated yeast cells. (*a* : × 11.200), (*b* : × 6.300), (*c* : × 9.750), (*d* : × 10.300).

C. albicans completely. This is due to the decline in functional capacity of the host cells in culture on the one hand and to the morphogenetic transformation of ingested *C. albicans* cells to germ tubes on the other. The germ tubes grow out of the host cells and develop into long branching hyphae which are too large to be handled further by the leucocytes. Moreover, leucocytes degenerate through their interactions with mycelial cells. Addition of ketoconazole in concentrations as low as $0.1\mu g/ml$ (a concentration which inhibits the outgrowth of hyphae from yeast phase cells and suppresses the growth of the remaining yeast cells) leads to complete elimination of the fungus (fig. 7). Some of the events taking place under the various conditions described above are shown in figures 8 to 15. This apparent synergism between the drug and the host-defence cells may explain, at least partly, the effectiveness of ketoconazole in eradicating deep fungal infections for continuous 'active' blood levels well above those that are growth and transformation inhibitory are achieved after a single daily dose (Brugmans et al., 1978). A similar co-culture set up with human and fungal cells provided semiquantitative data on the differential toxicity of a drug for the host cell and the pathogen (Aerts et al., 1980). In this system ketoconazole strongly inhibited the growth of *C. albicans* and some dermatophytes at a concentration of $10ng/ml$ while only being toxic for human fibroblasts at $100\mu g/ml$. The therapeutic ratio for ketoconazole in this system was thus 10^4. With the other imidazoles such as miconazole, econazole and clotrimazole this *in vitro* therapeutic margin is 10^2.

When the vaginas of rats artificially infected with yeast-phase *C. albicans*, were examined, beginning on the third day of infection, the predominant

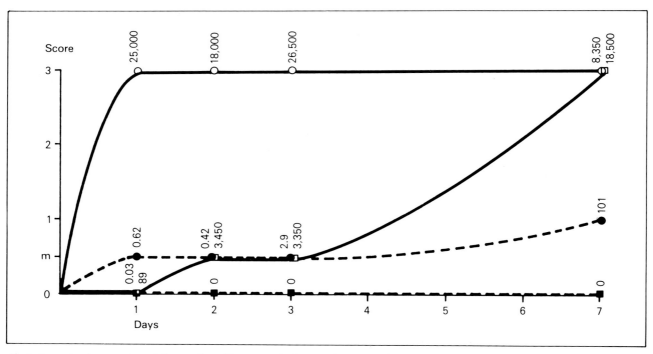

Fig. 7. Synergism between host defence cells and ketoconazole. Quantitative evaluation of the growth of *C. albicans*. The inocula were 450 yeast cells and 3×10^6 leucocytes. Ketoconazole was used at a concentration of $0.1\mu g/ml$. The points represent growth scores at the indicated times: — ○ — cultures of *C. albicans* only; ---●--- cultures of *C. albicans* treated with ketoconazole; —□— mixed cultures of *C. albicans* and leucocytes; ---■--- mixed cultures of *C. albicans* and leucocytes treated with ketoconazole. The figures on the graph give the corresponding numbers of colony forming units divided by 10^3. m = microscopically visible growth only (De Brabander et al., 1980).

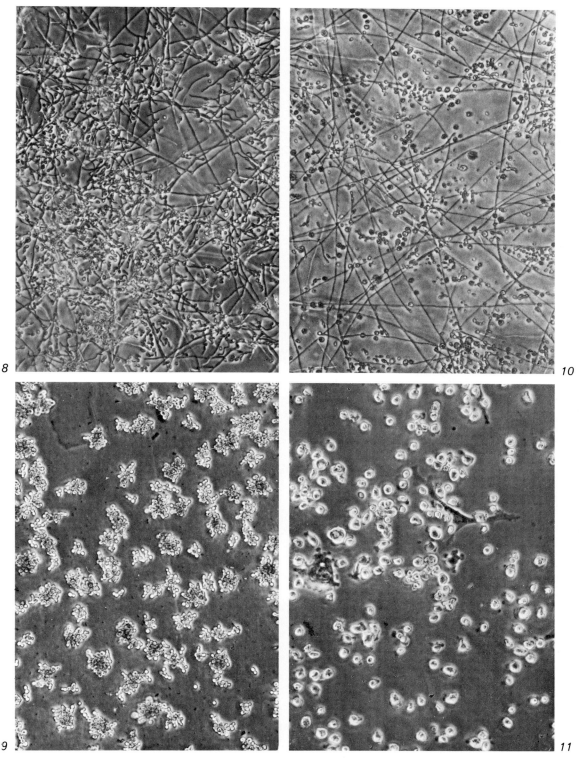

Synergism between host defence cells and ketoconazole. Phase contrast micrographs of cultures quantitated in figure 7.

Fig. 8. Culture of *C. albicans* after 2 days of growth. The mycelial form predominates. (× 115).

Fig. 9. Culture of *C. albicans* exposed to 0.1μg/ml ketoconazole and grown for 2 days. Only clusters of yeast cells are seen. (× 115).

Fig. 10. Mixed culture of *C. albicans* and leucocytes after 6 days of growth. Long branching mycelium predominates, the remaining leucocytes are necrotic. They are spherical and loosely attached to the hyphae. (× 115).

Fig. 11. Mixed culture of *C. albicans* and leucocytes exposed to 0.1μg/ml ketoconazole and grown for 6 days. Many viable and motile leucocytes are seen whereas *C. albicans* has been completely eradicated. (× 115).

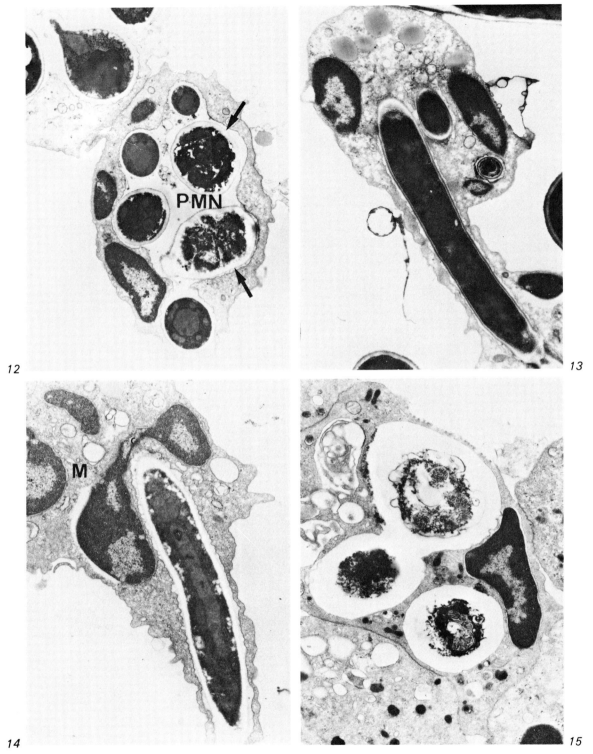

Synergism between host defence cells and ketoconazole

Fig. 12. Mixed culture of leucocytes and *C. albicans* after culture for 2h. The polymorphonuclear leucocyte (PMN) has engulfed 6 yeast cells of which only 2 (arrows) are killed. TEM (× 7.600).

Fig. 13. As figure 12, but after culture for 4h. An hypha grows out of the damaged leucocyte. TEM (× 7.600).

Fig. 14. As in figure 13, showing the growth of an hypha within a macrophage M. TEM (× 12.000).

Fig. 15. Mixed culture of leucocytes and *C. albicans* in the presence of 0.1μg/ml of ketoconazole, grown for 48h. The 3 yeast cells engulfed by a leucocyte are completely necrotic. TEM (X 11.200).

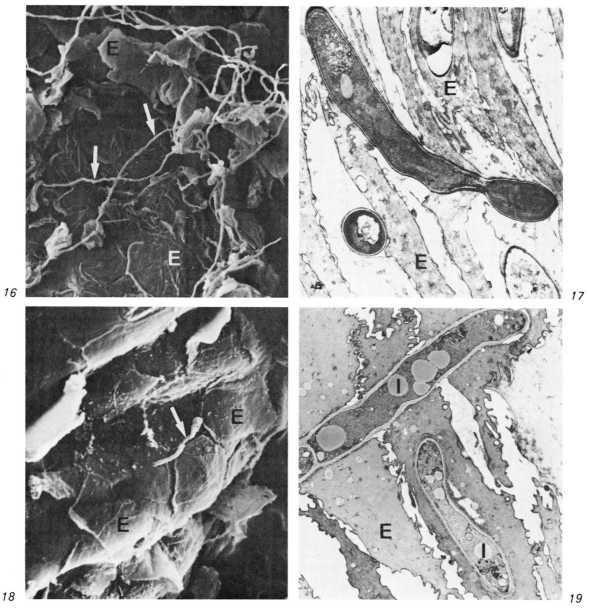

Experimental vaginal candidiasis in the rat

Fig. 16. Rat vagina 4 days after the infection with yeast phase *C. albicans.* Untreated. Note that the vaginal epithelial cells (E) are covered with numerous long branching mycelial cells (arrow). SEM (× 300).

Fig. 17. As in figure 16. This shows how a developing mycelial cell penetrates the keratinous epithelium (E). TEM (× 6.600).

Fig. 18. After 1 day of topical treatment with miconazole. An occasional hypha (arrow) remains at the epithelial surface (E). SEM (× 600).

Fig. 19. After 2 days of topical treatment with miconazole. Two necrotised hyphae, loaded with multiple lipid globules (1) are surrounded by unaltered epithelial cells (E). TEM (× 4.800).

morphogenetic form covering and invading the keratinous epithelial layers was the filamentous form (figs. 16-17). In a comparison of the efficiency of topical treatment of miconazole, clotrimazole and terconazole the very typical changes at the cell periphery occurred focally at altered hyphal branching points from the end of the first day of treatment. Most of the hyphae underwent necrosis by the second day of miconazole (figs. 18 and 19) and terconazole treatment, whereas a drastic reduction in the number of cells was seen after 3 days of treatment with clotrimazole (Van de Ven et al., 1980). Complete clearance of experimental vaginal candidiasis occurred with a 3-day treatment schedule of orally administered ketoconazole (Thienpont et al., 1980). The conclusions drawn from the comparative studies were that (1) there exists a direct correlation between the occurrence of drug related structural changes in *C. albicans* and the final cure rates of the animals; (2) the ultrastructural changes after *in vivo* challenge with the drugs are similar to those after *in vitro* exposure; (3) the order of *in vitro* fungitoxic potency is in agreement with *in vivo* order of potency of the 3 topically applied azole derivatives; (4) no abnormalities were induced in the surrounding vaginal epithelial cells with any of the topical treatment regimens.

Dermatophytoses: Inhibition of the filamentous fungi *Trichophyton mentagrophytes* and *Microsporum canis* after exposure to miconazole and ketoconazole has been shown to be accompanied by plasma membrane changes, similar to those seen with *C. albicans*. However, higher concentrations were needed to achieve these effects. Necrosis of the drug treated hyphae occurred after prolonged exposure to these drugs (Borgers, 1980). Scanning and transmission electron microscopic examination of skin scrapings of patients infected with *T. rubrum* revealed that very early after the onset of oral treatment with ketoconazole, the typical 'azole changes' in the cell wall and the internal necrosis of the hyphae occurred after 9 days of treatment (Degreef et al., in press). Examples of scanning and transmission electron microscopy of skin infected with *T. rubrum* and the effects of oral ketoconazole on the infected skin are shown in figures 20 to 23.

Deep mycoses: The alterations to the surface and internal structures of the various phases of *Coccidioides immitis* (Borgers et al., 1981), *Paracoccidioides brasiliensis* and *Histoplasma capsulatum* (Negroni de Bonvehi et al., 1980), *Cryptococus neoformans* and *Blastomyces dermatitidis* (unpublished results) induced by exposing cultures to ketoconazole and miconazole have been studied. In the case of *C. immitis*, the drugs inhibited the maturation of spherules into endospores, and again the typical azole derivative changes occurred in the walls of the maturing endospore entities of the spherules (figs. 24-29). This effect of the drugs might be of importance not only in controlling the spreading of the infection but in the final extermination of the organism as well. Miconazole and ketoconazole induced changes in the structure of mature, resting endospore cultures but aerobically growing endospores did not undergo necrosis during a 24-hour exposure. This indicates that spores of *C. immitis* are much less susceptible to these drugs than *C. albicans* cells. The transformation of arthroconidia of *C. immitis* into mycelium was fully prevented after treatment and the mycelial phase cells were most susceptible as substantial necrosis was induced within an exposure of 24 hours (figs. 30 and 31).

H. capsulatum and especially *P. brasiliensis* were found to be much more sensitive to ketoconazole than *C. immitis*. The observed ultrastructural

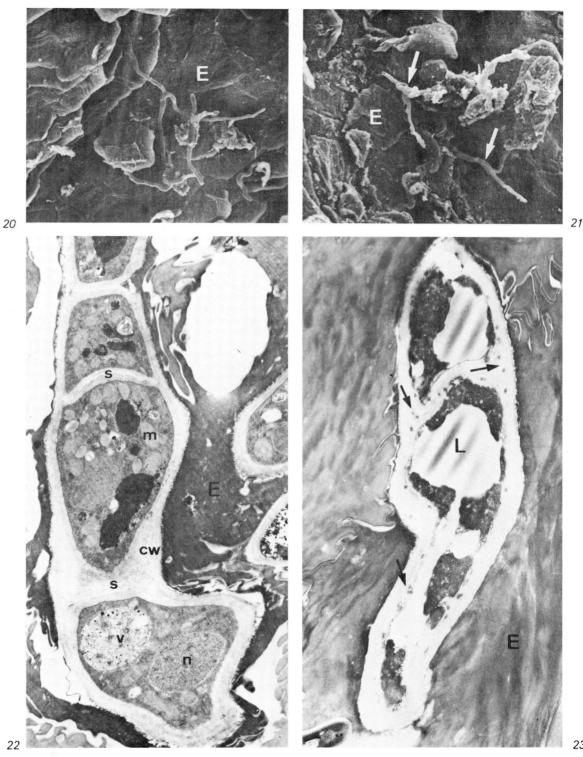

Trichophyton rubrum **in human skin**

Fig. 20. Pretreatment sample. Branching filaments covering and penetrating normal epithelial cells (E). SEM (× 500).

Fig. 21. After 9 days of oral medication with ketoconazole 200mg daily. Few altered hyphae remain. Note the collapsed appearance of the filamentous fungi (arrows). SEM (× 500).

Fig. 22. As in figure 20. Normal subcellular structures such as cell wall (cw), septae (s), nucleus (n), vacuole (v) and mitochondria (m) of *T. rubrum*, surrounded by the keratinous cell layers (E) are shown. TEM (× 11.00).

Fig. 23. As in figure 21. The necrotised hypha shows large cytoplasmic lipid globules (I) and multiple dense phospholipidic vesicles settle in the cell wall (arrows). TEM (× 20.000).

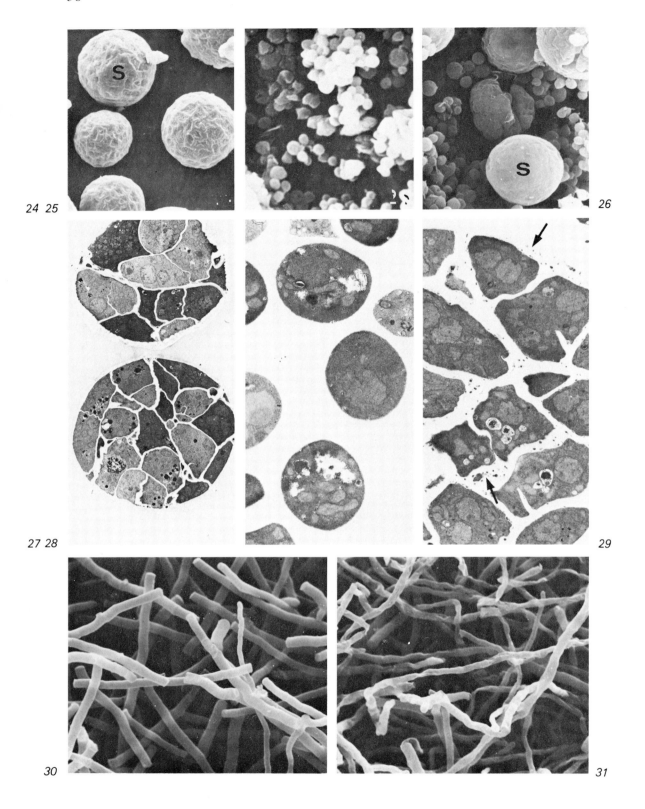

damage in both fungi resembled those in *C. albicans* exposed to keto-conazole and included surface changes, abnormal membrane prolifer-ation, fatty degeneration of the cytoplasm and lysis of subcellular organ-elles (figs. 32-35). Necrosis of *P. brasiliensis* was present at a concentra-tion of $0.1\,\mu g/ml$ but only after $1\,\mu g/ml$ in the case of *H. capsulatum* cells.

Although supported by preliminary observations only the structural damage brought about by these imidazoles to *C. neoformans* and *B. der-matitidis* closely resembles that seen in *H. capsulatum* (unpublished obser-vations).

Biochemical and Metabolic Changes in Imidazole Treated Microorganisms

Disturbance of permeability: The N- substituted imidazole derivatives clotrimazole (Iwata et al., 1973b; Yamaguchi and Iwata, 1979), econazole (Raab, 1980), imazalil (Siegel and Ragsdale, 1978) and miconazole (Van den Bossche, 1974; Sreedhara Swamy et al., 1970; Yamaguchi and Iwata, 1979; Dufour et al., 1980; Cope, 1980) alter membrane permeability of susceptible yeast and fungal cells. For example at concentrations as low as 10^{-9} to 10^{-8}M miconazole has been reported to inhibit the uptake of purines and glutamine by *C. albicans* and, at higher concentrations, to damage the cellular permeability barrier of this yeast causing leakage of inorganic cations, amino acids and proteins. Miconazole at about 5×10^{-5}M has an almost immediate effect on the exchange of intracellular potassium for extracellular protons across the cellular membrane of the yeast *Schizosaccharomyces pombe*. The effects described correlate well with morphological effects of low dose levels of for example miconazole, clotrimazole (De Nollin and Borgers, 1976; Borgers et al., 1979) and ketoconazole (Borgers et al., 1979).

The structural integrity and permeability of all cell membranes is largely determined by lipids (for reviews see: Brunner 1978; Lodish and Roth-man, 1979). Two kinds of lipid are included in membranes, cholesterol or another sterol and phospholipids. Cholesterol is found almost exclusively in the plasma membrane of mammalian cells, ergosterol is the main sterol found in yeast and fungal cells. Phospholipids are components of all biological membranes.

Effects on ergosterol synthesis: Both the morphological effects and alteration of membrane permeability might be, at least partly, a reflection of the effects of N-substituted imidazoles on ergosterol synthesis. In fact,

---

Coccidioides immitis **cultures**

Fig. 24. Untreated spherules. Inoculum. The surface of the large spherules (S) is slightly wrinkled. SEM ($\times$ 830).

Fig. 25. Untreated spherules after aerobic growth for 24h. All spherules matured into young endospores. SEM ($\times$ 830).

Fig. 26. After ketoconazole (10μg/ml). Aerobic growth for 24h. The development of endospores from spherules is suppressed. Altered spherules (S) remain. SEM ($\times$ 830).

Fig. 27. Same as figure 24. Section through a normal spherule. TEM ($\times$ 2.850).

Fig. 28. Same as figure 25. Normal young endospores are shown. TEM ($\times$ 10.000).

Fig. 29. Same as figure 26. The inhibited spherule presents characteristic phospholipid vesicles in the walls of the enclosed endospore entities (ar-rows). TEM ($\times$ 7.100).

Fig. 30. Untreated mycelium, aerobic growth for 24h. Long branching filaments possess a very smooth surface. SEM ($\times$ 975).

Fig. 31. Ketoconazole (10μg/ml). Aerobic growth for 24h. The large majority of the mycelium is collapsed. SEM ($\times$ 975).

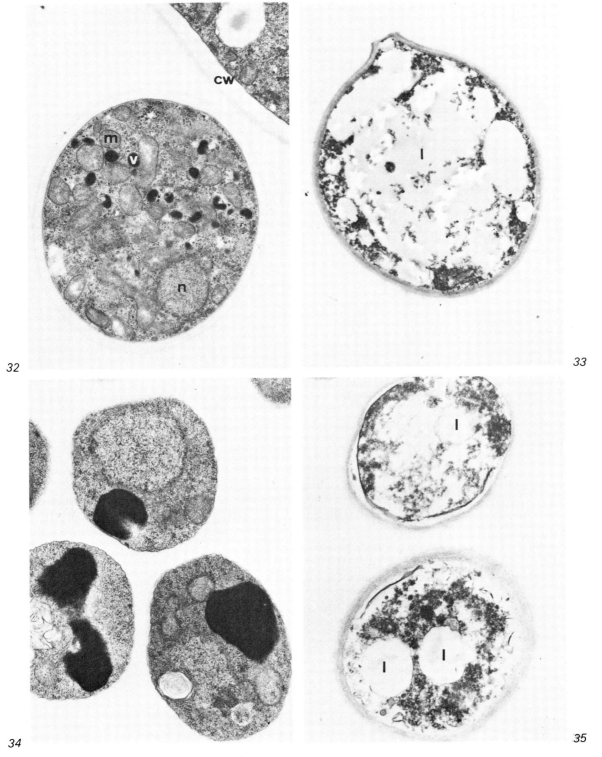

Paracoccidioides brasiliensis **yeast phase cells in culture**

Fig. 32. Untreated. The various organelles of this pathogen are shown. Mitochondria (m), nucleus (n), osmiophilic vesicles (v), cell wall (cw). (× 13.950).

Fig. 33. After ketoconazole (1μg/ml). The necrotic yeast cell is overloaded with lipid globules (l). (× 8.850).

Histoplasma capsulatum **yeast phase cultures**

Fig. 34. Untreated. Normal ultrastructure of 3 yeast phase cells (× 22.700).

Fig. 35. After ketoconazole (1μg/ml). Necrosis of the cytoplasm containing large lipid droplets (l) is seen in 2 cells (× 23.000).

Table I. Inhibition of ergosterol synthesis by imidazole and triazole derivatives

Drug	Species	References
Clotrimazole	*Candida albicans* *Ustilago avenae*	Haller (1978) Buchenauer (1978)
Imazalil	*Aspergillus nidulans* *Botrytis cinerea* *Penicillium expansum* *Ustilago maydis* *Ustilago avenae*	Siegel and Ragsdale (1978) Leroux and Gredt (1978) Buchenauer (1977)
Ketoconazole	*Candida albicans*	Van den Bossche et al. (1979) Van den Bossche et al. (1980)
Miconazole	*Candida albicans* *Ustilago maydis*	Van den Bossche et al. (1978) Henry and Sisler (1979)
Parconazole	*Candida albicans*	Van den Bossche (unpublished)
Terconazole	*Candida albicans*	Van den Bossche (unpublished)

as shown in table I, ergosterol synthesis is blocked by both imidazole and triazole derivatives in a great variety of species and strains of yeast and fungal cells. For example experimental evidence is available that ketoconazole is a potent inhibitor of ergosterol synthesis in *C. albicans* grown in culture media which support either yeast or mycelial growth. This inhibition occurred before any measurable effect on growth.

Interference of ketoconazole with ergosterol synthesis was also observed when the drug was added to cultures containing outgrown mycelium, a form mostly encountered *in vivo*. Furthermore, when administered to rats infected with *C. albicans* also, ketoconazole inhibits fungal synthesis of ergosterol. The dose influencing cholesterol synthesis by rat liver is 6 times that inhibiting ergosterol synthesis by microorganisms (Van den Bossche et al., 1980). Both imidazole derivatives affect sterol synthesis in subcellular fractions of *C. albicans*, *Saccharomyces cerevisiae* and rat liver. However, cholesterol synthesis in the subcellular fraction of liver is about 30 to 70 times less sensitive to ketoconazole or miconazole than ergosterol synthesis in a similar fraction obtained from both yeast cells (Willemsens et al., 1980).

Another reason for the *in vivo* selectivity of ketoconazole may be the dependence of yeast and fungi on their own ergosterol biosynthesis. Mammalian cells can utilise exogenous cholesterol from the diet and can compensate for the temporary effect of ketoconazole on cholesterol synthesis (Van den Bossche et al., 1979).

Accumulation of C-14 methylsterols: In all studies the inhibition of ergosterol synthesis coincides with an accumulation of sterols with a methyl group at C-14. In table II, sterols found in *C. albicans* grown in the absence and presence of ketoconazole are shown. The inhibition of ergosterol synthesis can thus be attributed to an interference with one of the reactions involved in the removal of the 14 α-methyl group of the precursor of ergosterol, lanosterol. Evidence is available that C-14 methyl

Table II. Sterols present in *C. albicans* grown in the absence and presence of ketoconazole

Ketoconazole	Sterols	
	C-14 desmethylsterols	C-14 methylsterols
−	Ergosterol, episterol	Lanosterol (trace)
+	−	14-Methylfecosterol, obtusifoliol, lanosterol, 24-methylenedihydrolanosterol

sterols, such as lanosterol, are unable to replace cholesterol or ergosterol in sterol-requiring cells (Nes et al., 1978; Bloch, 1979). For example *S. cerevisiae* kept under anaerobic conditions will grow in the presence of ergosterol whereas lanosterol does not sustain growth (Nes et al., 1978). Studies of Yeagle et al. (1977) on the effects of C-14 methyl sterols on properties of artificial membranes revealed that the presence of the 14 α-methyl is the principal feature responsible for the disparate membrane effects of lanosterol and for example cholesterol. By using glucose permeability as a parameter, it was shown that the incorporation of cholesterol into lecithin vesicles reduced the release of entrapped glucose from 50 to about 5%. However, when lanosterol replaced cholesterol in the vesicles, the release of trapped glucose from the vesicles resembled that occurring in the absence of cholesterol.

Based on these studies, it is reasonable to speculate that the presence of C-14 methyl sterols in yeast and fungal cells treated with azole derivatives may originate the permeability changes and inhibition of growth.

Effects on fatty acids, sterol esters, triglycerides and phospholipids: Alterations induced by the azole derivatives are not limited to an accumulation of lanosterol-like structures. At higher doses than those interfering with ergosterol biosynthesis, miconazole also intervenes in triglyceride and fatty acid synthesis (Van den Bossche et al. 1978).

Yamaguchi and Iwata (1979) reported that phospholipid liposomes are more sensitive to imidazoles when the acyl moieties are unsaturated. Sud et al. (1979) observed that the presence of unsaturated free fatty acids in liposome model membranes sensitised these membranes to the action of clotrimazole, miconazole and sulconazole. Yamaguchi (1978) also observed that the *in vitro* action of clotrimazole and miconazole was partly antagonised by the addition of phospholipids with unsaturated acyl moieties. This antagonistic effect might, among other things, be related with the recently observed miconazole induced shift from unsaturated to saturated acyl moieties of triglycerides, phospholipids and sterol esters and free fatty acids (Van den Bossche et al., unpublished). The acyl moiety of for example phospholipids and sterol esters from *C. albicans* grown in the presence of solvent, consisted of almost 50% of the unsaturated fatty acid, oleic acid, and respectively 16 and 13% of the saturated fatty acid, palmitic acid. However, after incubation for 16 hours in the presence of 5×10^{-8}M miconazole the phospholipids contained about 29% palmitic acid and 20% oleic acid. This shift is even more pronounced in the main phospholipid present in *C. albicans*, phosphatidyl choline (PC). In control cells PC contains almost 46% oleic acid and 7% palmitic acid but in cells treated with 10^{-8}M of miconazole the acyl moiety of PC consisted of 24% palmitate and 14% oleate. The acyl moiety of sterol esters extracted from *C. albicans* incubated for 16 hours in the presence of 5×10^{-8}M miconazole consisted of less than 15% oleic acid and of more than 45% palmitic acid. The fluidity of a membrane is determined not only by the sterols present, but also by the degree of saturation and chain length of the fatty acids of the phospholipid bilayer. The more unsaturated the fatty acids of membrane lipids are, the higher the permeability (De Gier, 1976). The greater amount of unsaturated fatty acids present the more active membrane fluidity and cellular growth are enhanced (Yamane and Tomioka, 1979). Therefore it is reasonable to speculate that the membranes of miconazole treated cells are more rigid than those of control cells and they will multiply more slowly.

The fluidity of a membrane not only determines the permeability (De Gier et al., 1971) but also the activity of some membrane-bound enzymes. For example the mitochondrial cytochrome *c* oxidase requires the fluid environment provided by unsaturated fatty acids (Vik and Capaldi, 1977).

Effects on oxidative and peroxidative enzymes: Miconazole at 0.5^{-5}µg/ml (10^{-6}-10^{-5}M) affects the membrane-bound enzymes cytochrome oxidase, NADH cytochrome *c* reductase and adenosine triphosphatase in *S. cerevisiae* (Van den Bossche, unpublished). Cytochrome *c* oxidase activity also decreased considerably after exposure of *C. albicans* to a fungistatic dose of miconazole (De Nollin et al., 1977). However, an increase of a cyanide insensitive NADH-dependent oxidase in the mitochondria and the central vacuolar system has been observed (Borgers et al. 1977). The oxidative pathway, of which the latter enzyme is part, leads to the production of hydrogen peroxide. Both miconazole (De Nollin et al., 1977) and ketoconazole (Borgers, 1980) block the cytochrome *c* peroxidase activity in the mitochondrial membranes of *C. albicans*. Simultaneously, the activity of catalase is enhanced. This increase is interpreted as a defence reaction to maintain low levels of intracellular peroxide. At higher doses of miconazole (> 5µg/ml), the NADH-dependent H_2O_2 production continues whereas the catalase becomes progressively inhibited. The hydrogen peroxide thus formed may contribute to the observed degeneration of subcellular structures that precedes cell death (Borgers, 1980).

The effects of imidazole derivatives on oxidative and peroxidative membrane-bound enzymes might be related to the observed structural changes of the acyl moieties in membrane lipids. However, many more studies are needed to understand this interrelationship.

Conclusion

Based on the effects induced by azole derivatives discussed here, the following hypothesis on the mechanism of action might be formulated:

Azole derivatives affect sterol metabolism in yeast or fungal cells resulting in an accumulation of 14 α-methylsterols known to disturb membrane and cell properties. Miconazole also influences the nature of fatty acids, free or esterified. The latter effect enhances the membrane disturbances, decreases growth and may lead to decreased activity of membrane-bound enzymes. It remains to be established whether there is any causative relationship between these events and the intracellular buildup of hydrogen peroxide observed on treatment with the azoles, which may contribute to cell death.

References

Aerts, F.; De Brabander, M.; Van den Bossche, H.; Van Cutsem, J. and Borgers, M.: The activity of ketoconazole in mixed cultures of fungi and human fibroblasts. Mykosen 23: 53-67 (1980).

Ansëhn, S.; Boquilt, L.; Schönebeck, J. and Winblad, B.: Effect of antimycotics on the surface morphology of Candida albicans. Castellania 2: 41-44 (1974).

Arai, T.; Mikami, T.; Yohoysma, K.; Kawata, T. and Naruda, K.: Morphological changes in yeasts as a result of the action of 5-fluorocytosine. Antimicrobial Agents of Chemotherapy 12: 255-260 (1977).

Bent, K.J. and Moore, R.H.: The mode of action of griseofulvin; in Biochemical Studies of Antimicrobial Drugs. 16th Symposium of Society of General Microbiology p.82-110 (Cambridge University Press, London 1966).

Bloch, K.: Speculations on the evolution of sterol structure and function. Critical Reviews in Biochemistry 7: 1-5 (1979).

Borelli, D.; Bran, J.L.; Fuertes, J.; Legendre, R.; Leiderman, E.; Levein, H.B.; Restrepo, M.A. and Stevens, D.A.: Ketoconazole, an oral antifungal: Laboratory and clinical assessment of imidazole drugs. Postgraduate Medical Journal 55: (1979).

Borgers, M.: Mechanism of action of antifungal drugs, with special reference to the imidazole derivatives. Review of Infectious Diseases 2: 520-534 (1980).

Borgers, M.; De Brabander, M. and Van den Bossche, H.: Differential effects of imidazole anti-fungal drugs on the yeast and mycelial phases of Candida albicans in vitro. Proceedings of the Royal Society of Medicine, International Congress and Symposium, Series Number 7: 21-23 (1979).

Borgers, M.; De Brabander, M.; Van den Bossche, H. and Van Cutsem, J.: Promotion of pseudomycelium formation of Candida albicans in culture: a morphologic study of the effects of miconazole and ketoconazole. Postgraduate Medical Journal 55: 687-691 (1979a).

Borgers, M.; De Nollin, S.; Thoné, F. and Van Belle, H.: Cytochemical localization of NADH oxidase in Candida albicans. Journal of Histochemistry and Cytochemistry 25: 193-199 (1977).

Borgers, M.; De Nollin, S.; Verheyen, A.; De Brabander, M. and Thienpont, D.: Effects of new anthelmintics on the microtubular system of parasites; in Borgers and De Brabander (Eds) Microtubules and Microtubule Inhibitors p.497-508 (North Holland, Amsterdam 1975).

Borgers, M.; Levine, H.B. and Cobb, J.M.: Ultrastructure of Coccidioides immitis after exposure to the imidazole antifungals miconazole and ketoconazole. Sabouraudia 19: 27-38 (1981).

Brugmans, J.; Scheygrond, H.; Van Cutsem, J.; Van den Bossche, H.; Baisier, A. and Hörig, Ch.: Orale Langzeitbehandlung von Onychomykosen mit ketoconazol. Mykosen 23: 405-415 (1980).

Brunner, G.: Struktur der Zellembran. Biologie in unserer Zeit 8: 65-74 (1978).

Buchenauer, H.: Mechanism of action of the fungicide imazalil in Ustilago avenae. Journal of Plant Diseases and Protection 84: 440-450 (1977).

Buchenauer, H.: Analogy in the mode of action of fluotrimazole and clotrimazole in Ustilago avenae. Pesticidal Biochemical Physiology 8: 15-25 (1978).

Cartwright, R.Y.; Shaldon, C. and Hall, G.H.: Urinary candidiasis after renal transplantation. British Medical Journal 2: 351 (1972).

Cope, J.E.: Mode of action of miconazole on Candida albicans. Effect on growth, viability and K^+-release. Journal of General Microbiology 119: 245-251 (1980).

D'Arcy, P.F. and Scott, E.M.: Antifungal agents; in Tucker (Ed) Progress in Drug Research, p.93-147 (Birkhäuser Verlag, Basel and Stuttgart 1978).

De Brabander, M.; Aerts, F.; Van Cutsem, J.; Van den Bossche, H. and Borgers M.: The activity of ketoconazole in mixed cultures of leukocytes and Candida albicans. Sabouraudia 18: 197-210 (1980).

De Gier, J.; Mandersloot, J.G.; Hupkes, J.V.; McElhaney, R.N. and Van Beek, W.P.: On the mechanism of non-electrolytes permeation through lipid bilayers and through biomembranes. Biochimica Biophysica Acta 233: 610-618 (1971).

De Gier, J.: Recent onderzoek aan modelsystemen; in Booij and Daems (Eds) Biomembranen 50 jaar na Gortel en Grendel, p.42-61 (Centrum voor Landbouwpublikaties en Landbouwdokumentatie, Wageningen 1976).

Degreef, H.; Van de Kerckhove, M.; Gevers, D.; Van Cutsem, J.; Van den Bossche, H. and Borgers, M.: Ketoconazole in the treatment of dermatophyte infections. International Journal of Dermatology (in press).

De Nollin, S. and Borgers, M.: The ultrastructure of Candida albicans after in vitro treatment with miconazole. Sabouraudia 12: 341-351 (1974).

De Nollin, S. and Borgers, M.: Scanning electron microscopy of Candida albicans after in vitro treatment with miconazole. Antimicrobial Agents and Chemotherapy 7: 704-711 (1975).

De Nollin, S. and Borgers, M.: An ultrastructural and cytochemical study of *Candida albicans* after *in vitro* treatment with imidazoles. Mykosen 19: 317-328 (1976).

De Nollin, S.; Van Belle, H.; Goossens, F.; Thoné, F. and Borgers, M.: Cytochemical and biochemical studies of yeast after *in vitro* exposure to miconazole. Antimicrobial Agents and Chemotherapy 11: 500-513 (1977).

Dufour, J.-P.; Bontry, M. and Goffeau, A.: Plasma membrane ATPase of yeast. Journal of Biological Chemistry 255: 5735-5741 (1980).

Evans, G. and White, N.H.: Effect of the antibiotics radicicolin and griseofulvin on the fine structure of fungi. Journal of Experimental Botany 18: 465-470 (1967).

Godefroi, E.G.; Heeres, J.; Van Cutsem, J.H. and Janseen, P.A.J.: The preparation and antimycotic properties of derivatives of 1-phenylethylimidazole. Journal of Medical Chemistry 12: 784-791 (1969).

Haller, I.: Imidazole-antimycotics: experience with clotrimazole, experimental aspects, aims for the future. p.56 Abstracts XII. International Congress of Microbiology, München (1978).

Hamilton-Miller, J.M.T.: Sterols from polyene-resistant mutants of *Candida albicans*. Journal of General Microbiology 73: 301-303 (1972).

Hamilton-Miller, J.M.T.: Chemistry and biology of the polyene macrolide antibiotics. Bacteriological Review 37: 166-196 (1973).

Heeres, J.; Backx, L.J.J.; Mostmans, J.H. and Van Cutsem, J.: The syntehsis and antifungal activity of ketoconazole, a new potent orally active broadspectrum antifungal agent. Journal of Medical Chemistry 22: 1003-1007 (1979).

Heeres, J., and Van den Bossche, H.: Antifungal chemotherapy; in Hess et al. (Eds) Annual Reports in Medicinal Chemistry, p.139-148 (Academic Press New York, 1980).

Henry, M.J. and Sisler, H.D.: Effects of miconazole and dodecylimidazole on sterol biosynthesis in *Ustilago maydis*. Antimicrobial Agents and Chemotherapy 15: 603-607 (1979).

Hoeprich, P.D.; Ingraham, J.L.; Kleker, E. and Winship, M.J.: Development of resistance to 5-fluorocytosine in *Cadida parapsilosis* during therapy. Journal of Infectious Diseases 130: 112-118 (1974).

Holt, R.J. and Newman, R.L.: The antimycotic activity of 5-fluorocytosine. Journal of Clinical Pathology 26: 167-174 (1973).

Iwata, K.; Kanda, Y.; Yamaguchi, H. and Osumi, M.: Electron microscopic studies on the mechanisms of action of clotrimazole on *Candida albicans*. Sabouraudia 11: 205-209 (1973a).

Iwata, K.; Yamaguchi, H. and Hiratani, T.: Mode of action of clotrimazole. Sabouraudia 11: 158-166 (1973b).

Janssen, P.A.J. and Van Bever, W.: Miconazole; in Goldberg (Ed) Pharmacological and Biochemical Properties of Drug Substances, 2: 333-345 (American Pharmacological Association, Washington 1979).

Kitajima, Y.; Sekiya, T. and Nozawa, Y.: Freeze-fracture ultrastructural alterations induced by filipin, pimaricin, nystatin and amphotericin B in the plasma membranes of *Epidermophyton, Saccharomyces* and red blood cells. A proposal of models for polyene-ergosterol complex-induced membrane lesions. Biochimica et Biophysica Acta 445: 452-465 (1976).

Kotler-Brajtbury, J.; Medeff, G.; Kobayashi, G.S.; Boggs, S.; Schleninger, D.; Pandey, R.C. and Rinehart, K.L., Jr.: Classification of polyene antibiotics according to chemical structure and biological effects. Antimicrobial Agents and Chemotherapy 15: 716-722 (1979).

Lampen, J.O.: Interference by polyenic antifungal antibiotics (especially nystatin and filipin) with specific membrane functions; in Biochemical Studies of Antimicrobial Drugs. 16th Symposium of Society of General Microbiology, p.111-130. (Cambridge University Press, London 1966).

Leroux, P. and Gredt, M.: Effets de quelques fongicides systémiques sur la biosynthèse de l'ergostérol chez *Botrytis cenerea* Pers., *Penicillium expansum* Link. et *Ustilago maydis* (DC) Cda. Annales de Phytopathologie 10: 45-60 (1978).

Levine, H.B. and Cobb, J.M.: Oral therapy for experimental coccidioidomycosis with R 41400 (ketoconazole), a new imidazole. American Review of Respiratory Diseases 118: 715-721 (1981).

Little, J.R.; Blanke, T.J.; Valeriote, F. and Medoff, G.: Immunoadjuvant and antitumor properties of amphotericin B; in Chirigos (Ed) Immune Modulations and Control of Neoplasia by Adjuvent Therapy, p.381-387 (Raven Press, New York 1978).

Lodish, H.F. and Rothman, J.E.: The assembly of cell membranes. Scientific American 240: 38-53 (1979).

Malawista, S.E.: Microtubules and the movement of melanin granules in frog dermal melanocytes. Annals of the New York Academy of Sciences 253: 702-710 (1975).

Malawista, S.E.; Sato, H. and Bensch, K.G.: Vinblastine and griseofulvin reversibly disrupt the living mitotic spindle. Science 160: 770-771 (1968).

Negroni de Bonvehi, H.B.; Borgers, M. and Negroni, R.: Ultrastructural changes produced by ketoconazole in the yeast-like phase of *Paracoccidioides brasiliensis* and *Histoplasma capsulatum*. Mycologia (In press).

Nes, W.R.; Sekula, B.C.; Nes, W.D. and Adler, J.H.: The functional importance of structural features of ergosterol in yeast. Journal of Biological Chemistry 253: 6218-6225 (1978).

Noguchi, T.; Kaji, A.; Igarashi, Y.; Shigematsue, A. and Taniguchi, K.: Anti-trichophyton activity of naphthiomates. Antimicrobial Agents and Chemotherapy 267: 2-9 (1962).

Norberg, B.: Cytoplasmic microtubules and radial segmented nuclei (Rieder cells). Effects of osmolality, ionic strength, pH, penetrating non-electrolytes, griseofulvin and a podophyllin derivative. Scandinavian Journal of Haematology 7: 445-454 (1970).

Odds, F.C.: Candida and candidosis. Monograph. Leicester University Press (1979).

Oxford, A.E.; Paistrick, H. and Simonart, P.: Studies in the biochemistry of microorganisms. LX. Griseofulvin $C_{18}H_{17}O_6Cl$, a metabolic product of *Penicillium griseofulvin* Dierckx. Biochemical Journal 33: 240-248 (1939).

Plempel, M.; Bartmann, K.; Buchel, K.H. and Regel, E.: BAY b 5097, a new orally applicable antifungal substance with broad-spectrum activity. Antimicrobial Agents and Chemotherapy 1969: 271-274 (1969).

Polak, A. and Grenson, M.: Evidence for a common transport system for cytosine, adenine and hypoxanthine in *Saccharomyces cerevisiae* and *Candida albicans*. European Journal of Chemistry 32: 276-282 (1973a).

Polak, A. and Grenson, M.: Interference between the uptake of pyrimidines and purines in yeasts. Pathological Microbiology 39: 37-38 (1973b).

Polak, A. and Scholer, H.J.: Fungistatic activity, uptake and incorporation of 5-fluorocytosine in *Candida albicans*, as influenced by pyrimidines and purines. I. Reversal experiments. Pathological Microbiology 39: 148-159 (1973a).

Polak, A. and Scholer, H.J.: Fungistatic activity, uptake and incorporation of 5-fluorocytosine in *Candida albicans* as influenced by pyrimidines and purines. Studies on distribution and incorporation. Pathological Microbiology 39: 334-337 (1973b).

Polak, A. and Scholer, H.J.: Mode of action of 5-fluorocytosine and mechanisms of resistance. Chemotherapia 21: 113-130 (1975).

Polak, A. and Scholer, H.J.: Mode of action of 5-fluorocytosine. Revue de l'Institut Pasteur de Lyon 13: 233-244 (1980).

Preusser, H.J.: Effects of *in vitro* treatment with econazole on the ultrastructure of *Candida albicans*. Mykosen 19: 304-316 (1976).

Raab, W.P.E.: The treatment of mycoses with imidazole derivatives. Monograph. (Springer-Verlag, Berlin 1980).

Robinson, H.M. and Raskin, J.: Tolnaftate, a potent topical antifungal agent. Archives of Dermatology 91: 372-376 (1965).

Shadomy, S.: *In vitro* studies with 5-fluorocytosine. Applied Microbiology 17: 871-877 (1969).

Shirley, S.F. and Little, J.R.: Immunopotentiating effects of amphotericin B. I. Enhanced contact sensitivity in mice. Journal of Immunology 123: 2878-2882 (1979a).

Shirley, S.F. and Little, J.R.: Immunopotentiating effects of amphotericin B. II. Enhanced *in vitro* proliferative responses of murine lymphocytes. Journal of Immunology 123: 2883-2889 (1979b).

Siegel, M.R. and Ragsdale, N.W.: Antifungal mode of action of imazalil. Pesticide Biochemistry and Physiology 9: 48-56 (1978).

Sreedhara Swamy, K.H.; Sirsi, M. and Ramanada Rao, G.: Studies on the mechanism of action of miconazole: effect of miconazole on respiration and cell permeability of *Candida albicans*. Antimicrobial Agents and Chemotherapy 5: 420-425 (1974).

Sud, I.J.; Chou, D.-L. and Feingold, D.S.: Effect of free fatty acids on liposome susceptibility to imidazole antifungals. Antimicrobial Agents and Chemotherapy 16: 600-663 (1979).

Symoens, J.; Moens, M.; Scheygrond, H.; Dony, J.; Schuermans, V.; Legendre, R. and Finestine, N.: An evaluation of two years of clinical experience with ketoconazole. Review of Infectious Diseases 2: 674-687 (1980).

Thienpont, D.; Van Cutsem, J. and Borgers, M.: Ketoconazole in experimental candidosis. Review of Infectious Diseases 2: 570-577 (1980).

Thienpont, D.; Van Cutsem, J.; Van Gerven, F.; Heeres, J. and Janssen, P.A.J.: Ketoconazole, a broad-spectrum orally active antimycotic. Experientia 35: 606 (1979).

Van Cutsem, J.; Zaman, R.; Van Gerven, F.; Thienpont, D. and Janssen, P.A.J.: Topical therapeutic treatment with R 42470 of vaginal candidosis, skin candidosis and dermatophytic infections in laboratory animals. Preclinical Research Report, Janssen Pharmaceutica, R 424701, Nr. 5 (1980).

Van den Bossche, H.: Biochemical effects of miconazole on fungi. I. Effects on the uptake and or utilization of purines, pyrimidines, nucleosides, amino acids and glucose by *Candida albicans*. Biochemical Pharmacology 23: 887-889 (1974).

Van den Bossche, H.; Cools, W.; Verheyen, A. and Vlaminckx, E.: Sensibilidad *in vitro* de Trichomonas vaginalis a miconazol y clotrimazol. Investigacion Medica International 7: 234-238 (1980).

Van den Bossche, H.; Willemsens, G.; Cools, W. and Cornelissen, F.: Inhibition of ergosterol synthesis in *Candida albicans* by ketoconazole. Archives Internationales de Physiologie et de Biochimie 87: 849-850 (1979).

Van den Bossche, H.; Villemsens, G.; Cools, W.; Cornelissen, F.; Lauwers, W.F. and Van Cutsem, J.M.: Effects of the antimycotic drug, ketoconazole, on sterol synthesis. An *in vitro* and *in vivo* study. Antimicrobial Agents and Chemotherapy 17: 922-928 (1980).

Van den Bossche, H.; Willemsens, G.; Cools, W.; Lauwers, W.F.J. and Lejeune, L.: Biochemical effects of miconazole on fungi. Inhibition of ergosterol biosynthesis in *Candida albicans*. Chemical and Biological Interactions 21: 59-78 (1978).

Van den Bossche, H.; Willemsens, G. and Van Cutsem, J.M.: The action of miconazole on the growth of *Candida albicans*. Sabouraudia 13: 63-73 (1975).

Van de Ven, M.; Borgers, M.; Thoné, F. and Van Custem, J.: Topical terconazole, miconazole and clotrimazole in experimental vaginal candidiasis. Janssen Pharmaceutica, Preclinical Research Report R 42479, Nr. 11 (1980).

Vik, S.B. and Capaldi, R.A.: Lipid requirements for cytochrome *c* oxidase activity. Biochemistry 16: 5755-5759 (1977).

Warner, J.F.; Duma, R.J.; McGehee, R.F.; Shadomy, S. and Utz, J.P.: 5-Fluorocytosine in human candidiasis. Antimicrobial Agents and Chemotherapy 1970: 473-475 (1971).

Weber, K.; Wehland, J. and Herzog, W.: Griseofulvin interacts with microtubules both *in vivo* and *in vitro*. Journal of Molecular Biology 102: 817-830 (1976).

Weinstein, M.J.; Oden, E.M. and Moss, E.: Antifungal properties of tolnaftate *in vitro* and *in vivo*. Antimicrobial Agents and Chemotherapy 595-601 (1964).

Willemsens, G.; Cools, W. and Van den Bossche, H.: Effects of miconazole and ketoconazole on sterol synthesis in a subcellular fraction of yeast and mammalian cells; in Van den Bossche (Ed) The Host Invader-Interplay, p.691-694, (Elsevier/North Holland Biomedical Press, Amsterdam 1980).

Woods, P.A.; Bard, M.; Jackson, I.E. and Drutz, D.J.: Resistance to polyene antibiotics and correlated sterol changes in two isolates of *Candida tropicalis* from a patient with an amphotericin B-resistant funguria. Journal of Infectious Diseases 129: 53-58 (1974).

Yamaguchi, H.: Protection of unsaturated lecithin against the imidazole antimycotics, clotrimazole and miconazole. Antimicrobial Agents and Chemotherapy 13: 423-426 (1978).

Yamaguchi, H. and Iwata, K.: Effect of two imidazole antimycotics clotrimazole and miconazole on amino acid transport in *Candida albicans*. Sabouraudia 17: 311-322 (1979).

Yamane, I. and Tamioka, F.: The concomitant effect of unsaturated fatty acid supplemented to medium on cellular growth and membrane fluidity of cultured cells. Cell Biology International Reports 3: 515-523 (1979).

Yeagle, P.L.; Martin, R.B.; Lala, A.K.; Lin, H.-K. and Bloch, K.: Differential effects of cholesterol and lanosterol on artifical membranes. Proceedings National Academy of Sciences USA 74: 4924-4926 (1977).

Chapter IV

Introduction to Antifungal Imidazoles

H.B. Levine

There have been excellent and detailed reviews in recent years on the anti-fungal imidazoles (Holt, 1976; Weinstein, 1978; Heel et al., 1980) but with few exceptions (Heeres and Van den Bossche, 1978; Borgers and Janssen, in press) these were written before the advent of extensive information on ketoconazole. The purpose of this overview is to provide an abbreviated background on the predecessors of ketoconazole and then to introduce ketoconazole's major properties *in vivo*, particularly its therapeutic efficacy in an animal model of severe coccidioidomycosis. Other papers in this volume will then describe the drug's advantages and limitations in managing a wide spectrum of fungal diseases in man.

That the imidazole family possesses antimicrobial properties was first shown clearly by Woolley (1944). He demonstrated that benzimidazole inhibited bacterial and fungal growth. The phenomenon was ascribed to competitive inhibition between the drug and adenine and guanine because of structural similarities among the 3 compounds and also because inhibitory activity could be reversed by purines. A very important contribution, and one that greatly influenced the pharmaceutical industry, was the finding of Jerchel et al. (1952) that the addition or alteration of substituent groups or atoms on benzimidazole influenced antimicrobial activity profoundly. During the subsequent quarter of a century a large number of substituted imidazole drugs were synthesised and tested for antifungal properties. A structural comparison of some of the more intensively studied antifungal imidazoles is shown in figure 1.

Seeliger (1958) reported that chlorimidazole inhibited a wide spectrum of fungi and Herrling et al. (1959) demonstrated additionally that this drug was of low toxicity. Other antifungals with relatively broad inhibitory spectrums include tioconazole, isoconazole and sulconazole; more restricted antifungal spectra are reported for thiabendazole (inactive against yeasts) and mebendazole. The principal compounds with clear and proven therapeutic value in man are clotrimazole, econazole, miconazole and ketoconazole. These, like most of the imidazoles, show *in vitro* inhibition of dermatophytes and yeasts at concentrations of 0.01 to 3μg/ml. Other imidazoles, including butoconazole, oxiconazole, democonazole and parconazole, have corresponding activity *in vitro* but for a variety of reasons have not been studied extensively in animal models or in human beings.

The mechanisms of action of the phenethyl imidazole compound miconazole have been studied extensively and are described in chapter III. In brief, like ketoconazole, it disrupts membrane function in *Candida albicans* without a polyene-like dependence on the presence of sterols in the fungal walls for disruptive activity to occur (Heeres and Van den Bossche, 1978; Milne, 1978; Hanifin, 1980; Van den Bossche et al., 1980; Borgers, 1980). Other inhibitory activities are mediated by interference with purine and glutamine uptake, and alteration of the organisms' peroxisome content and catalase function (De Nollin and Borgers, 1974; 1975). The resulting structural and ultrastructural damage and necrosis have been demonstrated also in fungi other than *Candida* (Borgers et al., 1981).

Miconazole was most effective when given by intravenous infusion or, in certain circumstances, into spinal fluid. The thrust of subsequent research was directed to the development of orally absorbed antifungal imidazoles. Dioxolane derivatives were studied in particular and many showed pro-

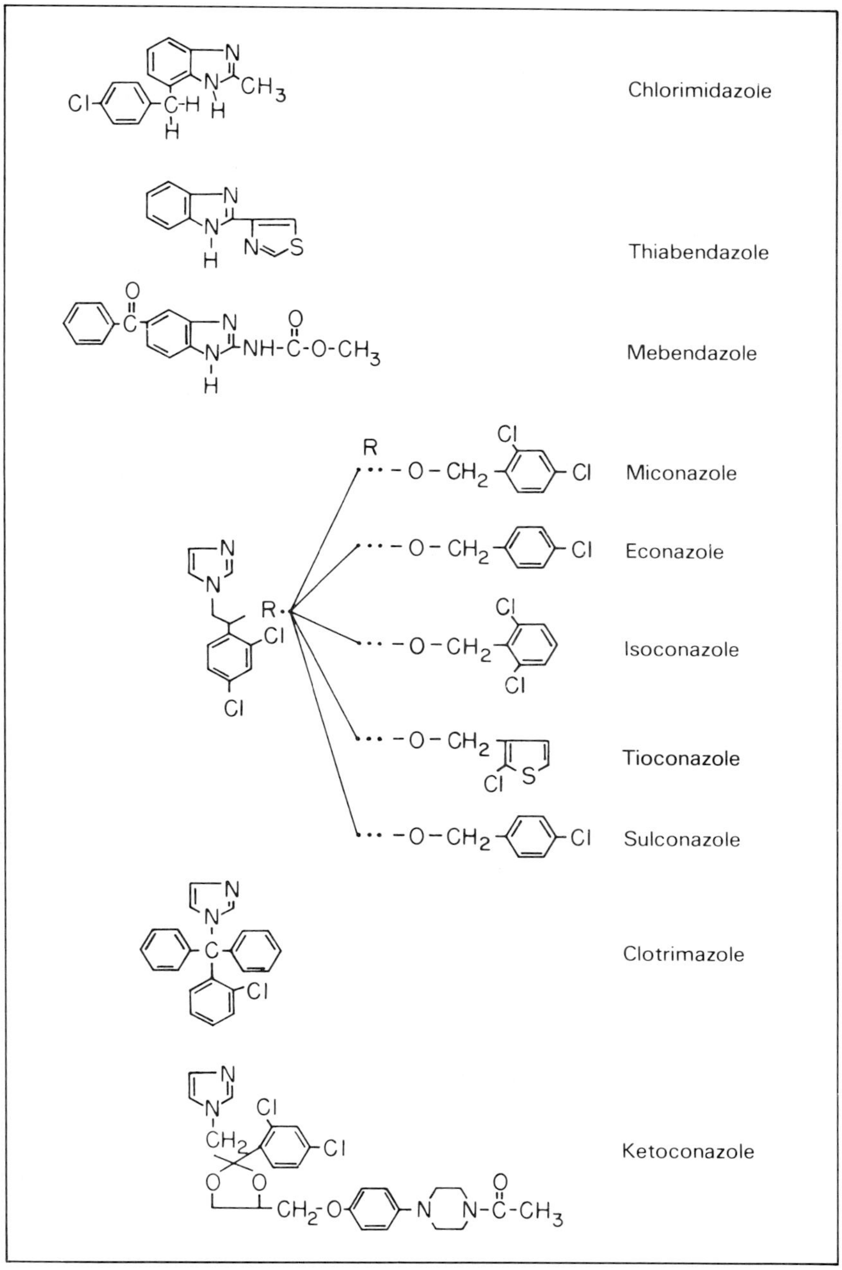

Fig. 1. The structures of selected antifungal imidazoles.

mise against *Candida* and dermatophytes (Van Cutsem and Thienpont, personal communication). Some, such as doconazole (Levine, 1976) and parconazole (Levine, unpublished) were active in experimentally produced deep mycotic disease. The trail led to ketoconazole which, as will be described in other chapters, was efficacious by the oral route in a broad spectrum of superficial and deep mycotic infections in humans and in animal models.

The pharmacology of ketoconazole has been studied extensively. Unlike miconazole, which has shown side effects in man (Medoff and Kobayashi, 1980), ketoconazole has a very low side effect profile (p.149). It is devoid of toxicity for bone marrow, peripheral blood, liver and kidney functions, serum electrolytes, calcium/phosphorus metabolism, bone formation, and ophthalmologic structure and function (p.76). In rats the dose of ketoconazole affecting cholesterol synthesis in the liver is about 6 times that dose which inhibits the fungal synthesis of ergosterol (Van den Bossche et al., 1980). The imidazoles as a class do not seem to induce significant resistance in susceptible organisms *in vitro* or during prolonged treatment (Levine et al., 1975; Levine and Cobb, 1978; Holt, 1975; Deresinski et al., 1977; Medoff and Kobayashi, 1980; Graybill and Drutz, 1980).

Prolonged use of ketoconazole does not induce hepatic enzymes interfering with anticoagulants or blood levels (p.73). The latter feature occurs during clotrimazole treatment; the induced enzymes mediate the degradation of clotrimazole (Holt, 1974), thus diminishing its therapeutic effectiveness. Because of this, and because of serious side effects (Kobayashi and Medoff, 1980), clotrimazole is used mainly as a topical antifungal agent. Ketoconazole has a biphasic decay with a 1.4 to 2.2 hour first phase half-life in man and a 7 to 10 hour second phase half-life (p.67). These are considerably longer than the decays for miconazole (Stevens, 1976) or econazole (Levine, 1978).

Initially miconazole and ketoconazole were developed primarily for the management of candidosis. The use of miconazole, and later ketoconazole, for deep mycotic infections, began with coccidioidomycosis after its efficacy had been demonstrated in animal models. But the studies in animals would have been unlikely to have been initiated had it not been for the observation of Dr Nardo Zaias of Miami, Florida, on a single patient who had been desperately ill with disseminated coccidioidomycosis, and had failed to respond to amphotericin B. Dr Zaias then turned to miconazole. The drug appeared to produce a rapid and dramatic improvement. The patient felt well and he refused further treatment after a short time. He soon returned, however, having relapsed into critical illness. After a second course of miconazole treatment, the patient again felt well and discontinued the medication. He then left Florida and was lost to follow-up.

Such changes in a patient's condition occur in coccidioidomycosis in the absence of treatment, as Dr Zaias recognised. But the changes experienced by this particular patient were very dramatic and impressed Dr Zaias to the extent that he persuaded others at the Naval Biosciences Laboratory in Oakland, California, to examine miconazole in a model system of pulmonary coccidioidomycosis in mice. The drug was clearly life-saving in all treated animals despite the use of infecting doses so severe that 90 to 100% of the nontreated animals succumbed (Levine et al., 1975). The *C. immitis* model system was incorporated into the screening procedure for miconazole and subsequent imidazole drugs (Levine, 1976; 1980; Levine and Cobb, 1978; 1980).

The model was employed in different stages of murine coccidioidomycosis: oral treatment with ketoconazole, administered shortly after intranasal infection of mice with arthrospores of *C. immitis,* was also life-saving, as it was with miconazole. Survival rates of 100% occurred at appropriate doses (table I). Additionally, and in contrast to miconazole, the drug prevented gross fungal colonisation of the peritoneal organs of most of the animals after they had been infected by the intranasal route.

This was the first indication that an imidazole had the capacity to prevent dissemination or to alter its course. And, as table I also shows, ketoconazole produced the first biological cures; 44 to 55 % of animals receiving early treatment became free of infection.

In these studies, treatments with ketoconazole were initiated on the fourth day of the infection. At this time, pulmonary lesions were young and the lesions still had a good blood supply (Levine, in press). The drug had an opportunity to reach loci of infection by the circulatory route. A more severe test of efficacy occurs if treatment is withheld for 13 days. In the resulting more advanced disease, the histological picture changes in murine coccidioidomycosis; the fungus is often found in caseous pulmonary lesions or in well-structured lesions having a very limited blood supply, and disseminated lesions in organs of the peritoneal cavity are prominent. Moribundity is apparent in many animals by the thirteenth day of the infection and deaths usually ensue by the fifteenth day. The results of an experiment where treatment was begun on the thirteenth day are shown in figure 2. The drug prevented death in all of 40 treated animals over a 4-week observation period; 38 % of the placebo treated control animals succumbed during this time. The treated animals were then maintained on ketoconazole therapy for 86 days with only 3 of the 40 dying. But in this model of treatment, initiated late in the course of the disease, only 8 % biological cures were obtained (data not shown).

Disseminated coccidioidomycosis in animals or man is difficult to treat. The data in table I illustrates the remarkable capacity of ketoconazole to preserve the life of infected animals. Other findings described in chapter XVI show parallel therapeutic advantages in human coccidioidomycosis. But in animals, as in man, eradication of the offending fungus in disseminated, deep-seated disease is often not achieved despite intense and prolonged treatment. This is not the case in other fungal infections, superficial and deep, where, as described later, biological cures are obtained frequently. Thus challenges have been met by ketoconazole, but challenges remain.

Table I. The influence of treatment with ketoconazole on mortality and the development of lesions in mice infected intranasally with arthrospores of *Coccidioides immitis*

Treatment	Dead/total	Coccidioidal lesions				No. of mice culture negative
		lung	liver	spleen	kidney	
No treatment	25/39	14/14	6/14	13/14	11/14	0
10mg/kg — od — day 4-21	8/10	10/10	4/10	10/10	6/10	0
20mg/kg — od — day 4-21	3/10	8/8	5/8	8/8	4/8	0
40mg/kg — od — day 4-21	0/10	10/10	3/10	10/10	4/10	0
30mg/kg — bid — day 4-50	0/6	6/6	5/6	1/6	0/6	0
40mg/kg — bid — day 4-50	0/14	10/14	4/14	7/14	0/14	1/14
80mg/kg — bid — day 4-50	0/9	5/9	0/9	2/9	0/9	5/9
80mg/kg — bid — day 4-100	0/9	1/9	0/9	0/9	0/9	4/9

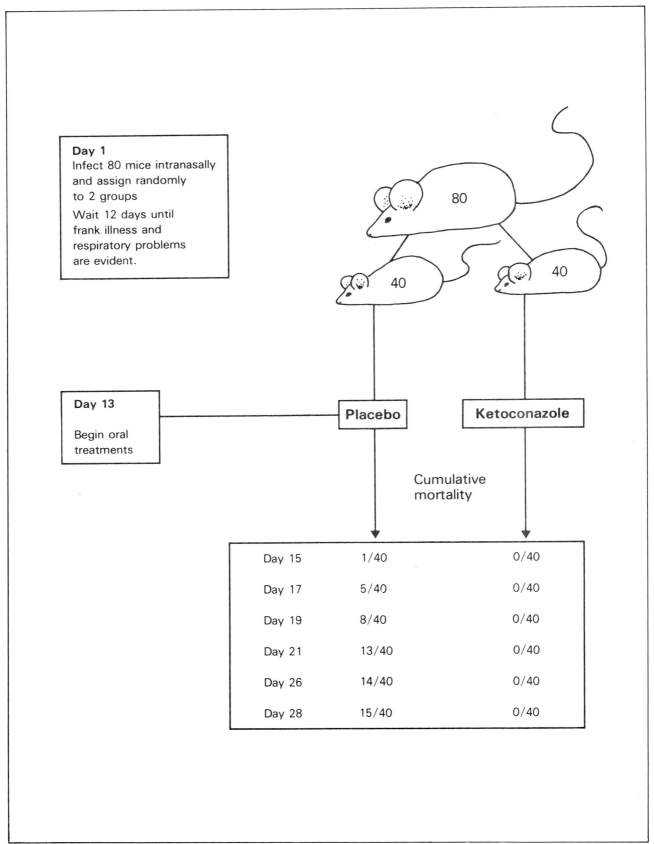

Fig. 2. Ketoconazole in advanced coccidioidal disease. The influence of delayed treatment with ketoconazole (35mg/kg twice daily) on mortality in mice infected intranasally with arthrospores of *Coccidioides immitis.*

References

Borgers, M.: Mechanism of action of antifungal drugs with special reference to the imidazole derivatives. Reviews of Infectious Diseases 2: 520-534 (1980).

Borgers, M.; Levine, H.B. and Cobb, J.M.: Ultrastructure of *Coccidioides immits* after exposure to the imidazole antifungals miconazole and ketoconazole. Sabouraudia 19: 27-38 (1981).

De Nollin, S. and Borgers, M.: The ultrastructure of *Candida albicans* after *in vitro* treatment with miconazole. Sabouraudia 12: 341-351 (1974).

De Nollin, S. and Borgers, M.: Scanning electron microscopy of *Candida albicans* after *in vitro* treatment with miconazole. Antimicrobial Agents and Chemotherapy 7: 704-711 (1975).

De Nollin, S. and Borgers, M.: An ultrastructural and cytochemical study of *Candida albicans* after *in vitro* treatment with imidazoles. Mykosen 19: 317-328 (1976).

Deresinski, C.; Galgiani, J.N. and Stevens, D.A.: Miconazole treatment of human coccidioidomycosis: Status report; in Ajello (Ed) *Coccidioidomycosis*. p.267-292 (Symposia Specialists, Miami 1977).

Graybill, J.R. and Drutz, D.J.: Ketoconazole: A major innovation for treatment of fungal disease. Annals of Internal Medicine 93: 921-923 (1980).

Hanifin, J.M.: Ketoconazole — an oral antifungal with activity against superficial and deep mycoses. Journal of American Academy of Dermatology 2: 537-539 (1980).

Heel, R.C.; Brodgen, R.N.; Pakes, G.E.; Speight, T.M. and Avery, G.S.: Miconazole: A preliminary review of its therapeutic efficacy in systemic fungal infections. Drugs 19: 7-30 (1980).

Herrling, S.; Sous, H.; Kruppe, E.; Osterloh, G. and Muckter, H.: Experimentelle Untersuchungen uber eine neue gegen Pilze Wirksame Verbindung. Arzneimittel-Forschung 9: 489-494 (1959).

Heeres, and Van den Bossche, H.: Antifungal chemotherapy; in Hess (Ed) Annual Reports in Medicinal Chemistry, p.139-148 (Academic Press, New York 1978).

Holt, R.J.: Recent developments in antimycotic chemotherapy. Infection 2: 95-107 (1974).

Holt, J.: Topical pharmacology of imidazole antifungals. Journal of Cutaneous Pathology 3: 45-59 (1976).

Jerchel, D.; Fischer, H. and Kracht, M.: Zur Darstellung der Benzimidazole. Liebigs Annalen der Chemie 575: 162-173 (1952).

Levine, H.B.: R34000, a dioxolone imidazole in the therapy for experimental coccidioidomycosis. Chest 70: 755-759 (1976).

Levine, H.B.: Econazole in experimental coccidioidomycosis. Current Chemotherapy 1: 233 (1978).

Levine, H.B.: Assay of antifungal drugs in experimental coccidioidomycosis. Proceedings Fifth Pan American Health Organsiation Symposium on Mycoses 396: 355-360 (1980).

Levine, H.B. and Cobb, J.M.: Oral therapy for experimental coccidioidomycosis with R41400 (ketoconazole), a new imidazole. American Review of Respiratory Diseases 118: 715-721 (1978).

Levine, H.B. and Cobb, J.M.: Ketoconazole in early and late murine coccidioidomycosis. Reviews of Infectious Diseases 2: 546-550 (1980).

Levine, H.B.; Stevens, D.A.; Cobb, J.M. and Gebhardt, A.E.: Miconazole in coccidioidomycosis. I. Assays of activity in mice and *in vitro*. Journal of Infectious Diseases 132: 407-414 (1975).

Medoff, G. and Kobayashi, G.S.: Strategies in the treatment of systemic fungal infections. New England Journal of Medicine 302: 145-155 (1980).

Milne, L.J.R.: The antifungal imidazoles: clotrizole and miconazole. Scottish Medical Journal 23: 149-152 (1978).

Seeliger, H.P.R.: Pilzhemmende Wirkung eines neuen Benzimidazole-Derivatives. Mykosen 1: 162-171 (1958).

Stevens, D.A.; Levine, H.B. and Deresinski, S.: Miconazole in coccidioidomycosis. II. Therapeutic and pharmacologic studies in Man. American Journal of Medicine 60: 191 (1976).

Van den Bossche, H.; Willemsens, G.; Cools, W.; Cornelissen, F.; Lauwers, F. and Van Cutsen, J.M.: *In vitro* and *in vivo* effects of the antimycotic drug ketoconazole on sterol synthesis. Antimicrobial Agents and Chemotherapy 17: 922-928 (1980).

Weinstein, J.: Current antifungal therapy; in Weinstein and Fields (Eds) Seminars in Infectious Disease, p.122-141 (Stratton, New York 1978).

Woolley, D.W.: Some biological effects produced by benzimidazole and their reversal by purines. Journal of Biological Chemistry 152: 225-232 (1944).

Ketoconazole:
Pharmacological Profile

Chapter V

In vitro and In vivo Activity

In vitro Antifungal Activity

Ketoconazole (research code R41,400; fig. 1) has a spectrum of antifungal activity *in vitro* which qualitatively resembles that of miconazole, an antifungal imidazole used topically or intravenously and, to a limited extent, orally. Quantitative results for minimum inhibitory concentrations of ketoconazole vary among laboratories, depending on inoculum size, culture medium, duration and temperature of incubation and growth phase of the fungus (Brass et al., 1979; Galgiani and Stevens, 1976; Granade and Artis, 1980; Grendahl and Sung, 1978; Holbrook and Kippax, 1979; Moody et al., 1978; unpublished data, on file Janssen Research Foundation). The results of *in vitro* tests are thus less relevant than *in vivo* studies, and may be misleading; it is noteworthy that for some conditions the impressive *in vivo* activity of ketoconazole could not have been predicted from commonly used *in vitro* tests. Nevertheless, *in vitro* testing provides a basic indication of the general spectrum of expected useful activity of an antifungal drug.

As illustrated in tables I and II, ketoconazole is active in the usual *in vitro* tests against a wide variety of dermatophytes, yeasts and other fungi. A recently developed *in vitro* model for *Candida albicans* (Borgers et al., 1979a,b) uses Eagle's minimal essential medium, a medium normally used to culture mammalian cells. In this model *C. albicans* grows rapidly and forms pseudomycelia, an interesting condition for evaluation of an

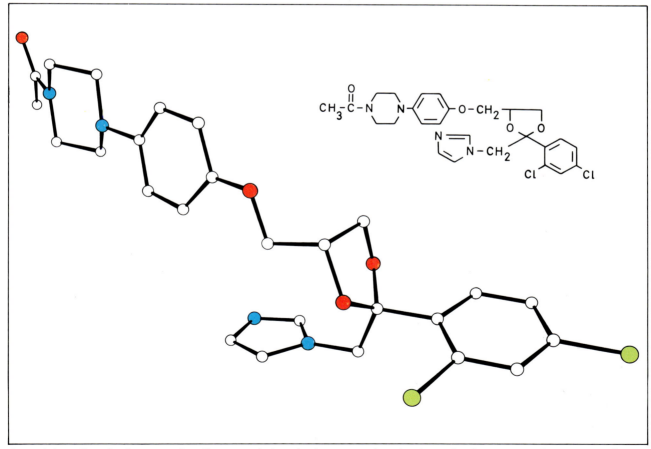

Fig. 1. A three-dimensional representation of ketoconazole drawn by the computer, based on the results of an x-ray crystallographic study (Peeters et al., 1979).

Table I. *In vitro* activity of ketoconazole against dermatophytes and yeasts

Organism	No. of strains tested	Range of minimal inhibitory concentrations (μg/ml)	References[1]
Dermatophytes			
Microsporum canis	24	0.1-64	a,b,c,d,e
Microsporum audouini	4	2-64	c,d
Microsporum gypseum	9	0.1-64	b,c,d
Microsporum cookei	1	1	b
Trichophyton mentagrophytes	24	0.1-20	a,b,c,d,e
Trichophyton rubrum	75	10^{-5}-128	a,b,c,d,e,f
Trichophyton ajelloi	1	1	b
Trichophyton schoenleini	1	1	b
Trichophyton tonsurans	35	0.25-16	b,c,d,e
Epidermophyton floccosum	23	0.1-8	b,c,d,e
Yeasts			
Candida albicans	472	0.02-80	a,b,d,f,g,h,i
Candida tropicalis	45	0.1-64	a,b,c,d,h
Candida pseudotropicalis	2	25-50	unpub.
Candida guilliermondii	4	0.4-50	unpub.
Candida krusei	14	0.2-3.1	h
Candida parapsilosis	18	0.2-64	a,b,c,f,g
Candida stellatoidea	1	0.8	unpub.
Cryptococcus neoformans	39	0.1-32	a,b,c,d,f,k,l
Torulopsis glabrata	124	0.8-64	a,b,c,f,g,d,h
Rhodotorula mucilanginosa	1	0.1	b
Trichosporon cutaneum	1	0.1	b

1 *References:* a = Heeres et al. (1979); b = Negroni (1977); c = Dixon et al. (1978); d = Holbrook and Kippax (1979); e = Grande and Artis (1980); f = Artis et al. (1981); g = Borelli et al. (1979); h = Moody et al. (1980); i = Polak (1980); j = Williams et al. (1980); k = Williams et al. (1979); l = Graybill et al. (1980); unpub. = unpublished data, on file Janssen Research Foundation. Unpublished data is also incorporated in some other instances.

antifungal drug since the predominant pathological form of *C. albicans in vivo* is the pseudomycelial form. When added to these well-developed but still growing mycelia, instead of the conventional yeast promoting media, ketoconazole was about 100 times more potent than miconazole in inhibiting pseudomycelial growth and causing subcellular changes, complete inhibition of pseudomycelial outgrowth occurring at concentrations of 5.3ng/ml and 0.48μg/ml with ketoconazole and miconazole, respectively.

Combining ketoconazole with other anti-infective agents *in vitro* usually does not produce increased antifungal activity, although synergism sometimes occurs *in vivo* with combination treatment (see below). Thus, a combination of ketoconazole and rifampin showed no evidence of synergism against *C. albicans* or *Torulopsis glabrata* (Moody et al., 1980), in contrast to the synergistic effect when miconazole and rifampin were combined. The *in vitro* susceptibility to ketoconazole of *Cryptococcus neoformans* and *Histoplasma capsulatum* is enhanced with the addition of amphotericin B, but is not altered when ketoconazole and flucytosine (5-fluorocytosine) are combined (Graybill et al., 1980).

The addition of 50% heat-inactivated pooled human serum to the culture medium increased by a factor of 20 the minimum inhibitory concentration of ketoconazole for *H. capsulatum,* and by a factor of 100 the minimum fungicidal concentration (Hawkins and Alford, 1980). Nevertheless, in the presence of serum ketoconazole remained fungicidal for *H. capsulatum* at concentrations $\leq 1\mu g/ml$.

In vitro Activity Against Other Organisms

Like other antifungal imidazoles, ketoconazole shows some activity *in vitro* against certain Gram-positive bacteria such as *Staphylococcus aureus, Staphylococcus epidermidis* or enterococcal streptococci, but it is less active in this regard than miconazole (Gaydos et al., 1979; Heeres et al., 1979).

Table II. *In vitro* activity of ketoconazole against dimorphic and other fungi

Organism	No. of strains tested	Range of minimal inhibitory concentrations ($\mu g/ml$)	References[1]
Dimorphic fungi			
Blastomyces dermatitidis	26	0.1-2	b,c,d,f,g
Coccidioides immitis	30	0.1-0.8	b,c,f,g,m,n,o
Histoplasma capsulatum	26	0.1-0.5	b,c,d,i,j,k,p
Paracoccidioides brasiliensis	5	0.002-0.1	b,f,g
Eumycetes			
Acremonium falciforme	1	10	b
Madurella grisea	1	0.1	b
Madurella mycetomi	1	0.1	b
Petriellidium boydii	23	0.1-4	b,c,d
Actinomycetales			
Actinomadura madurae	2	10-25	b,f,g
Nocardia asteroides	1	1	b
Nocardia brasiliensis	2	32-10	b
Nocardia cavea	1	1	b
Streptomyces sp.	1	10	b
Phycomycetes			
Absidia corymbifera	1	1	b
Rhizopus nigricans	1	100	b
Saprolegnia sp.	1	1	a
Various fungi			
Aspergillus flavus	2	1	b, unpub.
Aspergillus fumigatus	55	1-100	a,b,c,d
Aspergillus glaucus	1	1	b
Aspergillus nidulans	1	1	b
Aspergillus niger	6	1-16	b, unpub.
Aspergillus terreus	3	1	unpub.
Aspergillus spp.	3	5.5-100	f,g
Geotrichum candidum	1	1	b
Piedraia hortai	1	0.1	b
Sporothrix schenckii	23	0.1-16	a,b,c,d,f,g
Dematiacious fungi[2]	29	0.1-64	a,b,c,d

1   *References:* For key to a — l see table I. m = Levine and Cobb (1978); n = Levine and Cobb (1980); o = Levine and Cobb (1979); p = Hawkins and Alford (1980); unpub. = unpublished data, on file Janssen Research Foundation. Unpublished data is also incorporated in some other instances.
2   *Cladosporium* sp., *Fonsecaea* sp. and *Phialophora* sp.

Interestingly, ketoconazole has been shown to have *in vitro* activity against *Leishmania* at a high but potentially useful concentration (Berman, in press). Leishmaniasis is a significant problem in some parts of the world (e.g. Latin America, East Africa, parts of Asia and the Mediterranean area). Treatment has involved the use of parenteral agents such as antimony compounds, pentamidine or amphotericin B, which are difficult to administer under some conditions, and are potentially toxic and not always effective. An effective oral treatment for leishmaniasis would be a major advance, and the results of further studies with ketoconazole in this area will be awaited with interest.

At concentrations of 6 to 8μg/ml or greater ketoconazole also showed marked *in vitro* activity against both chloroquine-sensitive and chloroquine-resistant strains of *Plasmodium falciparum*, preventing parasite growth and producing morphological changes in existing parasites (Pfaller and Krogstad, 1980). No increase in parasite growth occurred in ketoconazole treated cultures in a 48-hour period after removal of the drug despite 8-hourly medium changes with drug-free medium.

Table III. Experimental fungal infections in which orally administered ketoconazole was effective

Experimental model	References[1]
Candidosis	
Systemic, in mice	Hatala et al. (1979); Polak (1980); Thienpont et al. (1980)
Systemic, in rats	Hatala et al. (1979)
Systemic, in guinea pigs	Thienpont et al. (1979, 1980)
Systemic, in rabbits	Unpub.
Systemic, in chickens	Thienpont et al. (1979, 1980)
Renal, in rats	Hatala et al. (1979)
Ocular, in rats	Green et al. (1979)
Gastrointestinal, in mice	Thienpont et al. (1980)
Gastrointestinal, in guinea pigs	Thienpont et al. (1980)
Crop, in turkeys	Thienpont et al. (1979, 1980)
Vaginal, in rats	Heeres et al. (1979); Thienpont et al. (1979, 1980)
Skin, in guinea pigs	Heeres et al. (1979); Thienpont et al. (1979, 1980)
Cryptococcosis	
Systemic, in mice	Graybill et al. (1980); unpub.
CNS, in rabbits	Perfect and Durack (1980)
Coccidioidomycosis	
Pulmonary, in mice	Borelli et al. (1979); Levine and Cobb (1978, 1980)
Blastomycosis	
Pulmonary, in mice	Borelli et al. (1979); Harvey et al. (1980)
Histoplasmosis	
Systemic, in mice	Graybill et al. (1980)
Dermatophytosis	
Skin, in guinea pigs	Thienpont et al. (1979); unpub.

1   Unpub. = unpublished data, on file Janssen Research Laboratories.

In vivo Activity

Orally administered ketoconazole has been effective in a wide variety of experimental yeast, dermatophyte and dimorphic fungus infections in various animal species (table III). In most such studies a daily dose of about 2.5 to 10 or 20mg/kg was needed for successful prophylaxis or treatment, although lethally challenged animals required higher doses [as did mice in whom ketoconazole may be less bioavailable than in man or other animal species (Graybill et al., 1980; unpublished data on file Janssen Research Foundation)].

Candidosis

Orally administered ketoconazole was effective prophylactically or therapeutically in animals with deep candidosis or vaginal or ocular infections (table IV). Although relatively high dosage levels were usually needed to markedly affect survival rates in 'normal' mice with systemic infections, in immunosuppressed mice a dosage of 10mg/kg/day improved the survival rate from 15% in controls to 55% (Hatala et al., 1979). An unpublished comparative study in mice infected intravenously with *C. albicans* showed ketoconazole at a dose of 160mg/kg/day given orally for 14 days to be more effective (6 of 7 animals surviving) than the same dose of miconazole, econazole or clotrimazole given orally (no survivors). It

Table IV. *In vivo* antifungal activity of orally administered ketoconazole in experimental candidosis

Experimental model, route of infection	Assessment criteria	Start of treatment relative to infection (hours)	Duration of treatment (days)[1]	Results [number of animals responding at dose levels (mg/kg/day) indicated][2]								References[4]
				0	2.5	5	10	20	40	80	160	
Mice, iv	survival	0	14	0/9		1/6	0/6	4/6	3/6	—	6/6	Unpub.
Mice, iv	survival	+ 24	7*	2/10			3/10	6/10	7/10	7/10		Unpub.
Mice, iv	survival	0	14*	7/20			20/20					a
Immunosuppressed mice, iv	survival	0	14*	3/20			11/20					a
Rats, kidney	survival	0	15	11/24			12/12	12/12	12/12			a
Rats, kidney	survival	+ 72	15	11/24			11/12	11/12	12/12			a
Rats, vaginal	cure	0	14	0/106	21/26	22/22						b,c
Rats, vaginal	cure	+ 72	3	0/62			3/6	83/85	6/6			b,c
Rats, vaginal	cure	+ 72	5*	0/17	1/5		27/30	18/18				b,c
Guinea pigs, iv	cure	− 24	14	0/15	4/6	6/11	15/15					b,c
Guinea pigs, dermal	cure	− 24	14	0/22	10/17		20/22					b,c
Rabbits, iv	survival	− 6	7	0/4							4/4[3]	Unpub.
Rabbits, iv	ocular lesions	+ 24	5	0/8						8/8		Unpub.
Chickens, iv	cure	0	14	0/18	3/6	6/6	12/12					b,c
Turkeys, crop	cure	0	13	0/18	16/22	13/14						b,c
Turkeys, crop	cure	+ 72	10	0/28	10/19	18/19	10/10					b,c

1 The drug was given as a single daily dose, except in those studies marked with an asterisk, where twice daily administration was used.
2 A shaded screen highlights the dosage for 100% response.
3 At a dose of 150mg/kg/day.
4 *References:* Unpub. = unpublished data, on file Janssen Research Foundation. Unpublished data is also incorporated in some other instances. a = Hatala et al. (1979); b = Thienpont et al. (1979); c = Thienpont et al. (1980).

was also slightly more effective than amphotericin B 0.25mg/kg/day intravenously or 160mg/kg/day orally (4 of 7 and 5 of 7 surviving, respectively), but was slightly less effective than amphotericin B in a higher intravenous dose (1mg/kg/day; 7 of 7 surviving).

In rats in which treatment was begun at the time of infection of the kidney with *Candida*, 100% survival was achieved with an oral dose of 5mg/kg/day (Hatala et al., 1979). Delaying treatment for 3 days increased the dose required for 100% survival to 20mg/kg/day.

Scanning electron microscope studies have demonstrated rapid disappearance of yeast cells from the infected vaginal tissue of ketoconazole treated rats, with complete eradication of the fungus after 5 days of treatment at an oral dose of 5mg/kg/day (Thienpont et al., 1980).

Cryptococcosis

At an oral dose of 86mg/kg/day for 16 days ketoconazole prolonged the life span of mice infected intravenously with *Cryptococcus neoformans* but did not prevent mortality. However, at a dose of 12mg/kg/day from days 3 to 17 after intraperitoneal infection the survival rate was increased to nearly 50%, compared with about 10% in controls (Graybill et al., 1980). In this study a combination of ketoconazole and amphotericin B (0.6mg 3 times weekly given intraperitoneally) was more effective than ketoconazole alone (over 90% survival with the combination) and was slightly more effective than amphotericin B alone (about 80% survival). In athymic (*nu/nu*) mice, which have severely impaired mechanisms of cell mediated immunity, neither drug alone significantly prolonged survival, but the combination did, despite eventual death in most even with combined therapy (less than 10% survival). When tissue cultures (spleen) were performed, a combination of ketoconazole (as above) and flucytosine (50mg/kg orally, twice daily) did not lower tissue counts more than with ketoconazole alone.

In immunosuppressed rabbits with experimental cryptococcal meningitis a combination of ketoconazole (200mg daily given orally) and amphotericin B (1mg/kg/day, intravenously) was superior to either drug given alone, and to a combination of amphotericin B and flucytosine (250mg daily given orally), as evaluated by cerebrospinal fluid culture 72 hours after infection (Perfect and Durack, 1980). By 2 weeks after infection both combination regimens had sterilised the cerebrospinal fluid.

Coccidioidomycosis

In mice infected intranasally with arthrospores of *Coccidioides immitis*, ketoconazole administered orally in doses of 10 and 20mg/kg/day, given once daily for 18 days starting on day 4 after infection, only slightly altered the disease course, but higher doses (40mg/kg once daily for 18 days to 80mg/kg twice daily for 96 days) prevented mortality and reduced the number of animals with liver, spleen or kidney lesions (Levine and Cobb, 1978, 1980). However, lung lesions were relatively resistant to treatment. When ketoconazole treatment was delayed after infection mortality was still reduced in treated animals compared with placebo (8% and 38% mortality with ketoconazole and placebo when treatment was started on day 12; 7% and 31% mortality when treatment was started on day 35), but some organ lesions persisted in most such animals (Levine and Cobb, 1980; fig. 2).

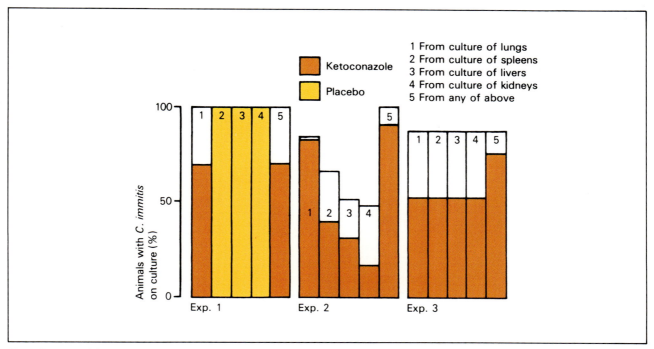

Fig. 2. Presence of fungi in organs of mice infected intranasally with *C. immitis*. Ketoconazole 35mg/kg twice daily was administered orally beginning on days 4 (exp. 1), 12 (exp. 2) or 35 (exp. 3) after infection (Levine and Cobb, 1980).

Blastomycosis

In experimental pulmonary blastomycosis in mice, oral administration of ketoconazole, 160mg/kg/day for 21 days, prevented mortality from a challenge lethal to 25% of the animals (LD_{25}) with *Blastomyces dermatitidis* (Borelli et al., 1979; Harvey et al., 1980). A dose of 80mg/kg/day prolonged survival but did not alter the eventual mortality rate after an LD_{90} challenge (Harvey et al., 1980). Intraperitoneal amphotericin B (6.25mg/kg/day) was completely protective in such animals.

Histoplasmosis

Ketoconazole (120mg/kg/day given orally on days 3 to 17 after infection) effectively protected mice from death following an intravenous challenge with *Histoplasma capsulatum*, 80% of treated mice surviving an otherwise lethal challenge (Graybill et al., 1980). Ketoconazole was more effective than amphotericin B given intraperitoneally (0.6mg 3 times a week; 50% survival), but a combination of the 2 drugs improved the response (about 90% survival) compared with ketoconazole alone. In *nu/nu* mice survival time was increased by treatment, but all animals eventually died.

Dermatophytosis

In guinea pigs with experimental skin infections with *Trichophyton mentagrophytes*, orally administered ketoconazole was markedly active at doses of 10mg/kg/day or higher. It was curative in all animals at a dose of 40mg/kg/day if treatment was begun 48 hours after infection and in 4 of 6 animals if begun 72 hours after infection. When *Microsporum canis* was the infecting organism lesion counts were markedly reduced at a dose of 40mg/kg/day, although some animals continued to show minimal lesions after 28 days of treatment. In a comparative study in *M. canis* infections, ketoconazole and griseofulvin, at the same dosage levels, produced similar results.

Development of Resistance

There is no evidence at present supporting the development of fungal resistance to ketoconazole or other imidazoles. Passage of *C. albicans* on agar layer plates containing increasing concentrations of ketoconazole seemed to slightly reduce the growth inhibitory effect of the drug (related to changes in sterol synthesis in the yeast cells) in some tests but not in others, depending on the culture method. When *in vitro* susceptibility testing was done before and after treatment, no development of resistance was shown by *C. albicans* isolated from the mouths of 4 patients treated for 2 weeks (200mg twice daily), or by *Coccidioides immitis* from mice after 17 days of treatment (Borelli et al., 1979; unpublished data, on file Janssen Research Foundation).

In a patient with chronic mucocutaneous candidosis receiving intermittent maintenance therapy with ketoconazole (200mg 3 times weekly) the minimum inhibitory concentration for the *Candida* increased during treatment (Rosenblatt et al., 1980). However, marked clinical improvement occurred with increased dosage (400mg daily). Whether this case represents development of resistance *per se,* or a tendency for long term therapy to 'select for' less sensitive strains, is not certain.

Conclusions

In vitro testing has shown ketoconazole to have the wide antifungal spectrum of other antifungal imidazoles such as miconazole. Interestingly, activity has also been demonstrated against *Leishmania* and *Plasmodium falciparum,* and these will be important areas for further study. In *in vivo* studies ketoconazole was active in a wide variety of experimental fungal infections in animals. Most noteworthy is that ketoconazole was effective on oral administration in all these animal models, whether the fungal infection was systemic or local.

References

Artis, W.M.; Odle, B.M. and Jones, H.E.: Griseofulvin-resistant dermatophytosis correlates with *in vitro* resistance. Archives of Dermatology 117: 16-19 (1981).

Berman, J.D.: Activity of imidazoles against *Leishmania tropica* in human macrophage en cultures. American Journal of Tropical Medicine and Hygiene (in press).

Borelli, D.; Bran, J.L.; Fuentes, J.; Leiderman, E.; Levine, H.B.; Restrepo-M, A. and Stevens, D.A.: Initial laboratory and multicenter clinical evaluation of R41 400, an oral antifungal. 18th Interscience Conference on Antimicrobial Agents and Chemotherapy, Atlanta, Georgia, 1-4 October (1978).

Borelli, D.; Fuentes, J.; Leiderman, E.; Restrepo-M, A.; Bran, J.L.; Legendre, R.; Levine, H.B. and Stevens, D.A.: Ketoconazole, an oral antifungal: laboratory and clinical assessment of imidazole drugs. Postgraduate Medical Journal 55: 657-661 (1979).

Borgers, M.; Van den Bossche, H.; De Brabander, M. and Van Cutsem, J.: Promotion of pseudomycelium formation of *Candida albicans* in culture: a morphological study of the effects of miconazole and ketoconazole. Postgraduate Medical Journal 55: 687-691 (1979a).

Borgers, M.; De Brabander, M.; Van den Bossche, H. and Van Cutsem, J.: The effects of the new antifungal ketoconazole on *Candida albicans;* in Kuttin and Baum (Eds) Proceedings of the XVIIth Congress of ISHAM (Excerpta Medica, Amsterdam 1979b).

Brass, C.; Shainhouse, J.Z. and Stevens, D.A.: Variability of agar dilution-replicator method of yeast susceptibility testing. Antimicrobial Agents and Chemotherapy 15: 763-768 (1979).

Dixon, D.; Shadomy, S.; Shadomy, H.J.; Espinel-Ingroff, A. and Kerkering, T.M.: Comparison of the *in vitro* antifungal activities of miconazole and a new imidazole, R41 400. Journal of Infectious Diseases 138: 245-248 (1978).

Galgiani, J.N. and Stevens, D.A.: Antimicrobial susceptibility testing of yeasts: a turbidimetric technique independent of inoculum size. Antimicrobial Agents and Chemotherapy 10: 721-726 (1976).

Gaydos, C.A.; Otey, C.S.; Brown, S.L.; Keiser, J.F. and Fischer, G.W.: Susceptibility of staphylococcus and enterococcus to miconazole and ketoconazole. Presented at the American Society for Microbiology Annual Meeting, Los Angeles, California (1979).

Granade, T.C. and Artis, W.M.: Antimycotic susceptibility testing of dermatophytes in microcultures with a standardized fragmented mycelial inoculum. Antimicrobial Agents and Chemotherapy 17: 725-729 (1980).

Graybill, J.R.; Williams, D.M.; Van Cutsem, E. and Crutz, D.J.: Combination therapy of experimental histoplasmosis and cryptococcosis with amphotericin B and ketoconazole. Reviews of Infectious Diseases 2: 551-558 (1980).

Green, M.T.; Broberg, P.H.; Jones, D.B. and Gentry, L.O.: Efficacy of oral ketoconazole in experimental endogenous Candida endophthalmitis. 11th International Congress of Chemotherapy, 19th Interscience Conference on Antimicrobial Agents and Chemotherapy, Boston (1979).

Grendahl, J.G. and Sung, J.P.: Quantitation of imidazoles by agar-disk diffusion. Antimicrobial Agents and Chemotherapy 14: 509-513 (1978).

Harvey, R.P.; Isenberg, R.A. and Stevens, D.A.: Molecular modifications of imidazole compounds: Studies of activity and synergy *in vitro* and of pharmacology and therapy of blastomycosis in a mouse model. Reviews of Infectious Diseases 2: 559-569 (1980).

Hatala, M.; Modr, Z. and Liska, M.: Oral treatment of experimental candidosis with R41 400 (ketoconazole). 11th International Congress of Chemotherapy and 19th Interscience Conference on Antimicrobial Agents and Chemotherapy, Boston, Massachusetts, 1-5 October (1979).

Hawkins, S. and Alford, R.: Human serum inhibition of ketoconazole activity against *Histoplasma capsulatum* in liquid culture. Presented at the 20th Interscience Conference on Antimicrobial Agents and Chemotherapy, New Orleans, Louisiana, 22-24 September (1980).

Heeres, J.; Backx, L.J.J.; Mostmans, J.H. and Van Cutsem, J.: Antimycotic imidazoles. Part 4. Synthesis and antifungal activity of ketoconazole, a new potent orally active broad-spectrum antifungal agent. Journal of Medicinal Chemistry 22: 1003-1005 (1979).

Holbrook, W.P. and Kippax, R.: Sensitivity of *Candida albicans* from patients with chronic oral candidiasis. Postgraduate Medical Journal 55: 692-694 (1979).

Levine, H.B. and Cobb, J.M.: Oral therapy for experimental coccidioidomycosis with R41 400 (ketoconazole), a new imidazole. American Review of Respiratory Diseases 118: 715-721 (1978).

Levine, H.B. and Cobb, J.M.: Therapy for experimental coccidioidomycosis with ketoconazole. Models for acute and chronic diseases. Proceedings of the 24th Annual Coccidioidomycosis Study Group Meeting, Las Vegas, Nevada, 15 May (1979).

Levine, H.B. and Cobb, J.M.: Ketoconazole in early and late murine coccidioidomycosis. Reviews of Infectious Diseases 2: 546-550 (1980).

Moody, M.R.; Schimpff, S.C.; Morris, M.J.; Young, V.M. and Wiernik, P.H.: *In vitro* activity of miconazole, miconazole nitrate, and R41 400 alone and combined with rifampin against *Candida* spp. and *Torulopsis glabrata* recovered from cancer patients. Presented at the 18th Interscience Conference on Antimicrobial Agents and Chemotherapy, Atlanta, Georgia, 1-4 October (1978).

Moody, M.R.; Young, V.M.; Morris, M.J. and Schimpff, S.C.: *In vitro* activities of miconazole, miconazole nitrate, and ketoconazole alone and combined with rifampin against *Candida* spp. and *Torulopsis glabrata* recovered from cancer patients. Antimicrobial Agents and Chemotherapy 17: 871-875 (1980).

Negroni, R.: Accion antifungica de nuevos compuestos imidazolicos. Actas de las VIII Jornadas y Primer Congreso Argentina de Micologia, Cordoba, 4-8 de Octubre (1977).

Peeters, O.M.; Blaton, N.M. and De Ranter, C.J.: Cis-1-acetyl-4-(4-[/2-(2,4-dichlorophenyl)-2-(1H-1-imidazolyl-methyl)-1,3-dioxolan-4-yl/]methoxy]phenyl)-piperazine: Ketoconazole a crystal structure with disorder. Acta Crystallographica B35: 2461 (1979).

Perfect, J.R. and Durack, D.T.: Comparison of amphotericin (AMB), 5-fluorocytosine (5FC) and ketoconazole (KTZ) in treatment of experimental cryptococcal meningitis. Interscience Conference on Antimicrobial Agents and Chemotherapy, New Orleans, Louisiana, September (1980).

Pfaller, M.A. and Krogstad, D.J.: Activity of ketoconazole against chloroquine-resistant plasmodium falciparum *in vitro*. Abstract. American Society for Clinical Investigation (1980).

Polak, A.: Determination de la synergie entre la 5-fluorocytosine et trois derives de l'imidazole au moyen de differents modeles *in vitro* et *in vivo*. Bulletin De La Societe de Mycologie Medicale 9: 263-268 (1980).

Rosenblatt, H.M.; Byrne, W.; Ament, M.E.; Graybill, J. and Stiehm, E.R.: Successful treatment of chronic mucocutaneous candidiasis with ketoconazole. Journal of Pediatrics 97: 657-660 (1980).

Thienpont, D.; Van Cutsem, J.; Van Gerven, F.; Heeres, J. and Janssen, P.A.J.: Ketoconazole — a new broad spectrum orally active antimycotic. Experientia 35: 606 (1979).

Thienpont, D.; Van Cutsem, J. and Borgers, M.: Ketoconazole in experimental candidosis. Reviews of Infectious Diseases 2: 570-577 (1980).

Williams, D.M.; Graybill, J.R. and Drutz, D.J.: Ketoconazole therapy of murine cryptococcosis and histoplasmosis. 11th International Congress of Chemotherapy and 19th Interscience Conference on Antimicrobial Agents and Chemotherapy, Boston, Massachusetts, 1-5 October (1979).

Williams, D.M.; Graybill, J.R.; Drutz, D.J. and Levine, H.B.: Suppression of cryptococcosis and histoplasmosis by ketoconazole in athymic nude mice. Journal of Infectious Diseases 141: 76-80 (1980).

Chapter VI

Pharmacokinetic Properties

Assay Methods

For the measurement of ketoconazole in biological material, gas, liquid and high performance liquid chromatographic methods and a bioassay have been developed (Andrews et al., 1981; unpublished data, on file Janssen Research Foundation). The chromatographic assays are specific for unchanged ketoconazole. The gas chromatographic method has an overall recovery of about 90 %, with minimum detectable concentrations below 0.01 µg/ml (plasma and urine) or 0.01 µg/g (faeces and tissues). The high performance liquid chromatographic method has a maximum sensitivity of about 0.1 µg/ml. The bioassay, based on *in vitro* inhibition of the growth of *Candida albicans,* is practical and reliable, but is less sensitive than the gas chromatographic method; minimum detectable concentrations are 0.05 µg/ml (or µg/g). The results obtained with the chromatographic methods and the bioassay are comparable.

Absorption and Elimination in Animals

Absorption in Animals

Absorption of tritiated ketoconazole from the gastrointestinal tract is more rapid in rats and guinea pigs (maximum plasma concentrations at 0.25 to 1 hour) than in rabbits and dogs (maximum concentrations at 1 to 2 hours). Following a dose of 10 mg/kg peak plasma concentrations were 1.0, 3.7, 8.9 and 16.5 µg/ml in rabbits, guinea pigs, dogs and rats, respectively. The extent of absorption was approximately similar in fasted and non-fasted rabbits, although peak concentrations were slightly lower but occurred slightly sooner in fasted animals. In rats a sex-related difference in the rate of absorption was seen, absorption occurring more rapidly in males (peak concentrations at 0.25 to 1 hour and 1 to 4 hours in males and females, respectively). Areas under the plasma concentration-time curves (AUC) vary more than 10-fold among species given the same dose, the largest AUC's occurring in dogs and rats.

Metabolism in Animals

In dogs and rats ketoconazole is extensively metabolised into a large number of inactive metabolites. Major metabolic pathways in these species include oxidation and subsequent scission and degradation of the imidazole ring, scission and degradation of the piperazine ring, scission of the dioxolane ring and oxidative-*O*-dealkylation. No antifungal activity was detectable in urine and bile samples or extracts in these animals.

Excretion in Animals

After 24 hours male rats had excreted 90 % of the radioactivity from a single tritiated dose of ketoconazole (10 mg/kg) given orally, and females about 78 %. Within 4 days both sexes excreted more than 95 % of the administered radioactivity. Similarly, female dogs eliminated about 80 % of administered radioactivity within 48 hours and 92 % within 7 days. In both male and female rats the elimination half-life ($t_{1/2\beta}$) was about 26 hours.

Male rats excreted 17 % of the radioactivity in the urine, and females 5 %. Biliary excretion accounted for the majority of a dose in rats, with 60 % eliminated in the bile after 24 hours. In female dogs urine accounted for about 9 % of administered radioactivity, and faeces about 83 %. A higher proportion of unchanged drug was recovered from the faeces of dogs (55 %) than from the faeces of rats (4 to 6 %).

Absorption and Elimination in Man

Absorption in Man

In healthy subjects, a single oral dose of ketoconazole 200 mg as a tablet containing the free base produced peak plasma concentrations of about 3 to 4.5 µg/ml at 1 to 2 hours after administration. Higher and more consistent plasma levels were reached when ketoconazole was taken with a meal. Prior treatment with cimetidine markedly reduced the oral absorption of ketoconazole, particularly when the stomach acidity was further reduced by the administration of bicarbonate (Van Der Meer et al., 1980). Since ketoconazole is lipophilic (log $P = 3.73$ in octanol/water), its bioavailability is higher and more consistent when it is administered with or just before a meal. Since it is a dibasic compound the acidity of the stomach plays an important role; ketoconazole requires sufficient gastric secretion for dissolution and subsequent absorption.

In healthy volunteers given increasing doses in tablet form, as well as a solution of ketoconazole as a reference, just before breakfast, the areas under the concentration-time curves correlated closely with peak plasma concentrations (figs. 1 and 2). Figure 1 illustrates the similar absorption pattern for the 200mg tablet as compared with the solution, although the relative bioavailability of the tablet was slightly lower (about 75%). As suggested by figure 2, ketoconazole may undergo 'first pass' metabolism during the absorption phase, with transient saturation of the metabolising capacity of the liver.

Metabolism and Excretion in Man

Four days after an oral dose of tritiated ketoconazole administered to 3 healthy males 70% of the dose had been excreted, about 57% in the faeces and 13% in the urine. Following absorption ketoconazole was extensively metabolised; unchanged drug accounted for 20 to 65% of the faecal radioactivity but for only 2 to 4% of urinary radioactivity. In the 0 to 24 hour urine, 30 to 50% of the metabolites were basic compounds, 5 to 10% polar acidic compounds and 5 to 10% conjugates of polar acidic compounds. About 35% of the urinary metabolites could not be extracted. In faecal methanol extracts basic metabolites accounted for more than 80% of the radioactivity. The various metabolites in the urinary and faecal extracts were separated and purified by high-performance liquid chromatography and the major metabolites analysed by mass spectrometry. The main identified metabolic pathways were oxidation of the imidazole ring, degradation of the oxidised imidazole, oxidative O-dealkylation, oxidative degradation of the piperazine ring and aromatic hydroxylation.

In healthy subjects the elimination half-life ($t_{1/2\beta}$) of ketoconazole was 6.5, 8.1 and 9.6 hours after a single oral dose (given as a tablet) of 100, 200 and 400mg, respectively.

Pharmacokinetics in Patients with Renal Impairment

In a small number of patients with severe renal failure absorption of ketoconazole occurred more slowly, and peak plasma concentrations were lower than in healthy subjects, but such differences were not statistically significant and the overall extent of absorption did not differ between the two groups. As might be expected, in the patients with renal insufficiency urinary excretion of unchanged ketoconazole was minimal (0.06% compared with 0.3% in healthy subjects), but in both groups this form of elimination was clinically unimportant. Thus, it appears that dosage adjustments in patients with renal impairment will not be required with ketoconazole. In a preliminary study on a few patients with some evidence of liver dysfunction, ketoconazole plasma concentrations were not altered compared with other subjects; however, further studies will be needed before any effects of liver disease on ketoconazole disposition can be adequately evaluated.

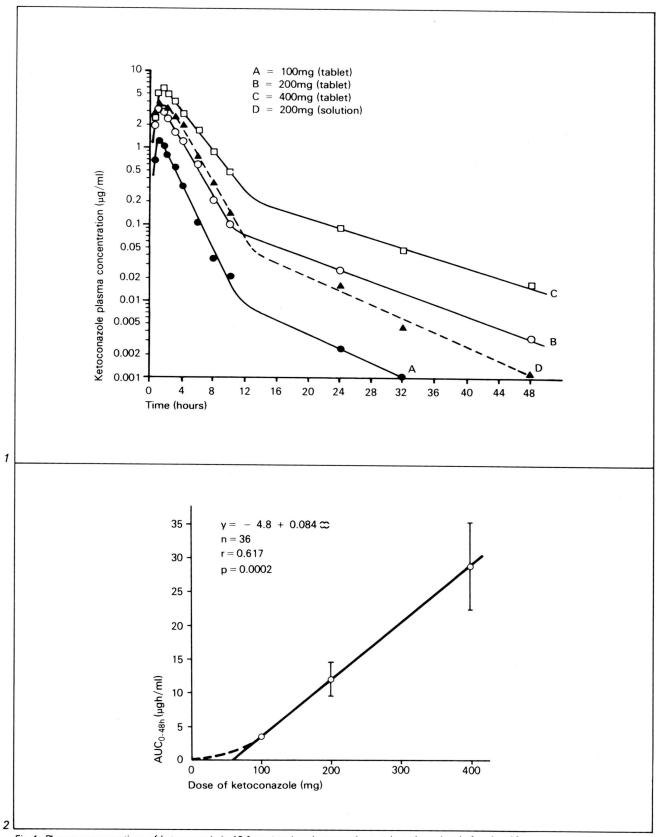

Fig. 1. Plasma concentrations of ketoconazole in 12 fasted male volunteers given various doses just before breakfast.

Fig. 2. Mean area under the plasma concentration-time curves after ketoconazole administration, as in figure 1.

(Unpublished data, on file Janssen Research Foundation).

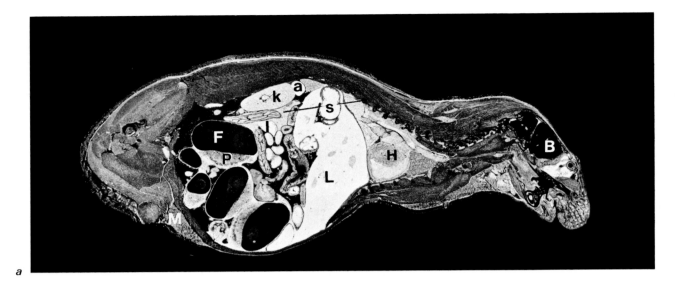

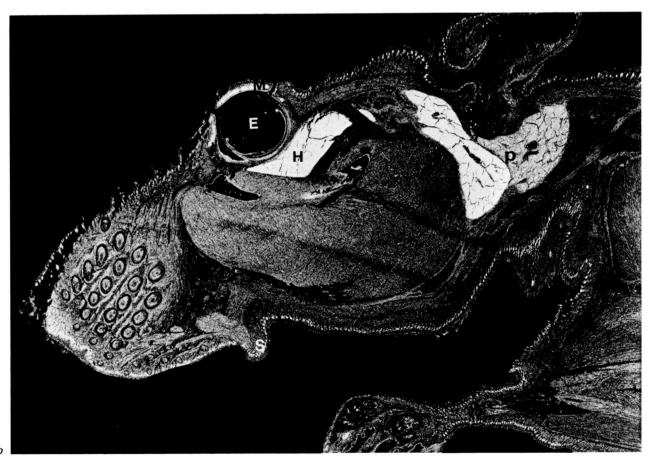

Fig. 3. Whole-body autoradiographs showing the deposition of ketoconazole in (a) the pregnant rat, 1 hour after dosing, and (b) the male rat, 8 hours after dosing, with orally administered H³-ketoconazole 20mg/kg. White areas represent high levels of radioactivity. (Fig. 3a: a = adrenal; B = brain; F = fetus; H = heart; I = intestine; k = kidney; L = liver; P = placenta; s = stomach. Fig. 3b: E = eyeball; H = Harder's gland; M = Meibomian (tarsal) gland; P = parotid; S = sebaceous glands.)

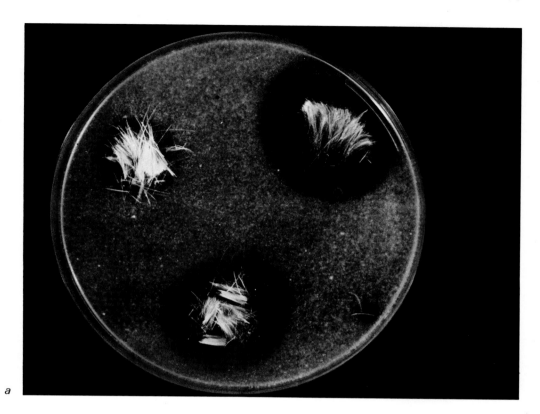

a

Fig. 4. Antifungal activity (bioassay with Trichophyton mentagrophytes). Guinea pig hairs 8 hours (fig. 3a) and 48 hours (fig. 3b) after a single oral dose of ketoconazole 40mg/kg (Van Cutsem et al., 1980). In each figure the sample in the 10 o'clock position is hair nearest the skin, in the 2 o'clock position is a 'middle' hair sample and in the 6 o'clock position is outer hair.

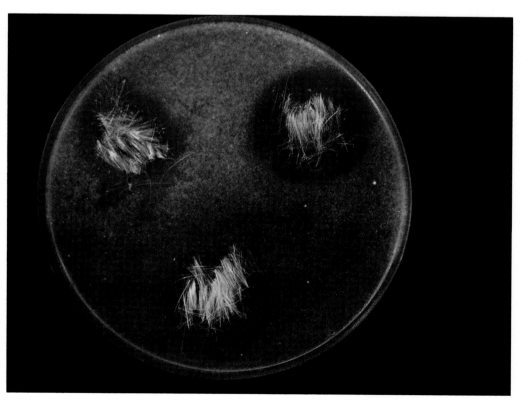

b

Distribution to Body Tissues

Tissue Distribution in Animals

Following a single oral dose of tritiated ketoconazole 20mg/kg given to rats, highest tissue levels of radioactivity occurred in the liver (125µg/g) and the adrenals (93 and 156µg/g in males and females, respectively), with moderate levels in the lung, kidney, bladder, bone marrow, teeth, myocardium and various glandular tissues. Marked distribution to connective tissue was noted. Lowest tissue levels occurred in the testis and brain; peak levels in the brain (2.3 to 2.7µg/g) were about one-tenth of the corresponding plasma concentrations. Radioactivity was also spread throughout the subcutaneous tissue (fig. 3). The fur of both rats and guinea pigs shows persistent antifungal activity after ketoconazole administration (fig. 4) and it has been suggested that the drug may be excreted with sebum (Van Cutsem et al., 1980).

Ketoconazole reached the placenta and uterus of pregnant rats given a single oral dose of 20mg/kg of tritiated drug on day 18 of gestation, about 0.8% of the administered dose appearing in each of these tissues (fig. 3a). Maximum fetal tissue concentrations occurred after 2 hours, amounting to about 0.5% of the dose. However, fetal concentrations were much lower than placental levels, indicating relatively poor penetration of the placental barrier. Similarly, in pregnant guinea pigs studied by whole body autoradiography ketoconazole or its metabolites crossed into the placenta slowly, but fetal tissue concentrations were markedly lower than maternal tissue levels.

Tissue Distribution in Man

In man a single oral dose of 200mg given to healthy subjects produced detectable concentrations of ketoconazole in urine, saliva, sebum and cerumen. In a few patients with various deep mycoses (whether any had fungal meningitis is unclear) peak cerebrospinal fluid concentrations of 2µg/ml and 7µg/ml occurred 3 to 4 and 1 to 2 hours after doses of 200 and 400mg, respectively. Concentrations of 1µg/ml or more persisted for 5 to 6 hours (unpublished data, on file Janssen Research Foundation). In a patient with candidal meningitis receiving ketoconazole 400mg twice daily, peak cerebrospinal fluid concentrations of 3.0 and 2.2µg/ml occurred 6 and 8 hours after a 400mg dose, following 7 days and 30 days of therapy, respectively (Fibbe et al., 1980). These cerebrospinal fluid concentrations corresponded with plasma levels of 9.5 and 9.0µg/ml. Thus, it appears that like other available antifungal imidazoles cerebrospinal fluid

Table I. Peak serum concentrations after ketoconazole 200mg and clinical response in patients with various superficial or deep mycoses

Type of mycosis	Peak serum concentration[1]		
	< 1µg/ml	1-4µg/ml	> 4µg/ml
Superficial	13/13 (100%)	53/60 (88%)	10/13 (77%)
Deep	1/4 (25%)	40/55 (73%)	6/15 (40%)
All	14/17 (82%)	93/115 (81%)	16/28 (57%)

1   Results shown as number of responders/total, with percentage response in parentheses.

penetration of ketoconazole is relatively low, but concentrations which might be expected to be effective against many fungal pathogens may be achieved.

Plasma Concentration and Clinical Effects

There is no correlation between peak serum concentrations achieved after a single dose of ketoconazole and clinical response (table I). Routine monitoring of ketoconazole serum concentrations during treatment would seem to be of little value.

Effect on Microsomal Enzymes

The effect of a systemically absorbed drug on hepatic microsomal enzymes is of interest from several perspectives, including the potential for drug interactions with other drugs metabolised in the liver, the likelihood of the drug stimulating its own metabolism (as occurs with clotrimazole) and the possibility of ultrastructural changes within the liver. Compounds which alter drug metabolism often exert a biphasic effect, with initial inhibition of drug metabolism on acute administration followed by stimulation of metabolism after about 12 hours (Conney, 1967). On acute administration ketoconazole, like econazole, miconazole and clotrimazole, produced some initial inhibition of drug metabolism in animal models (methohexitone sleep time, nicoumalone prothrombin time), but only at relatively high doses. Of the drugs tested only clotrimazole showed evidence of microsomal induction with repeated administration. It therefore seems that ketoconazole is unlikely to alter hepatic drug metabolising capacity to an important extent.

Conclusions

Ketoconazole is well absorbed from the gastrointestinal tract, achieving plasma concentrations after oral administration that should be clinically useful in many fungal infections. However, tissue concentration would provide a better indication of expected usefulness in many conditions; further studies are needed to define and quantify more clearly the tissue distribution of ketoconazole in man. Other areas requiring clarification include the effect of disease states (particularly liver disease) on the disposition of ketoconazole, and the relationship, if any, between plasma (or tissue) concentration and clinical effectiveness, although preliminary evidence suggests that a close relationship between plasma concentration and therapeutic results may not exist.

References

Andrews, F.A.; Peterson, L.R.; Beggs, W.H.; Crankshaw, D. and Sarosi, G.A.: Liquid chromatographic assay of ketoconazole. Antimicrobial Agents and Chemotherapy 19: 110-113 (1981).

Conney, A.H.: Pharmacological implications of microsomal enzyme induction. Pharmacology Reviews 19: 317-366 (1967).

Fibbe, W.E.; Van Der Meer, J.W.M.; Thompson, J. and Mouton, R.P.: CSF concentrations of ketoconazole. Journal of Antimicrobial Chemotherapy 6(5): 681 (1980).

Van Cutsem, J.; Van der Flaes, M.; Thienpont, D.; Dony, J. and Hörig, Ch.: Quantitative bestimmung von ketoconazol in den haaren oral behandelter ratten and meerschweinchen. Mykosen 23(8): 418-425 (1980).

Van Der Meer, J.W.M.; Keuning, J.J.; Scheijgrond, H.W.; Heykants, J.; Van Cutsem, J. and Brugmans, J.: The influence of gastric acidity on the bio-availability of ketoconazole. Correspondence. Journal of Antimicrobial Chemotherapy 6(4): 552-554 (1980).

Chapter VII

Toxicology and Safety Studies

Animal Toxicity

The lethal single dose for one-half of the animals (LD_{50}) of various species receiving ketoconazole orally or intravenously is shown in table I.

In rats and dogs treated for periods of 3 to 12 months with orally administered ketoconazole, no changes occurred with doses up to 10mg/kg/day.

Daily doses of 20 and 40mg/kg given in the diet to Wistar rats produced slight changes, which were accentuated at higher doses of 80 or 160mg/kg/day. Death occurred in 2 of 20 female rats at the 80mg/kg dose level and in 2 of 10 males at 160mg/kg. Signs of toxicity included reduced food consumption and weight gain, but little change in behaviour, appearance or haematological parameters. Gross pathology and histopathology showed changes in the liver, kidney, adrenals and ovaries, reflected in increased serum sodium and blood urea nitrogen concentrations and reduced serum potassium, urinary creatinine and urinary specific gravity. A tendency to increased bone fragility in female rats, possibly related to anoestrus, was noted. However, all fractures were secondary to manipulation, and no evidence of osteoporosis was present on x-ray or histopathological examination.

In Beagle dogs the liver was even more clearly the primary target of toxicity. At a daily dose of 40mg/kg of ketoconazole for 1 year (administered as a capsule) no deaths occurred, but appetite was reduced with emesis and decreased weight gain. Liver weight was increased, with increased serum concentrations of glutamic-pyruvic transaminase (SGPT) and alkaline phosphatase, and lipofuscin formation and deposition evident on histopathological examination. At a dose of 60mg/kg/day for 20 weeks more marked increases in SGPT and alkaline phosphatase concentrations occurred, along with increased liver weight and reduced weight of the thymus. However, all such changes were reversible on discontinuation of treatment. At a dose of 80mg/kg daily changes as above occurred, as well as severe gastritis, jaundice and death after 2 to 4 weeks.

Effects on Reproduction

Doses of up to 80mg/100g of food (about 80mg/kg/day) in male rats and up to 40mg/100g in female rats had no effect on fertility. At a dose of 80mg/100g of food in females the pregnancy rate was reduced. In peri- and postnatal studies a high dose in the food (160mg/100g) produced a low pregnancy rate with small litter sizes and fewer live fetuses. Pups were small at birth and failed to gain weight, most dying within a few days. Administered by gavage, a dose of 10mg/kg/day was without effects, but at 40mg/kg/day maternal toxicity occurred and 50% of fetuses were born dead, the remainder dying soon after birth. At a dose of 80mg/kg/day by gavage no fetuses were born alive.

Table I. LD_{50} (mg/kg) for ketoconazole 7 days after administration of a single dose

Species	Intravenous administration		Oral administration	
	male	female	male	female
Mice	46.6	41.5	786	618
Rats	85.9	85.9	287	166
Guinea pigs	23.3	32.5	178	226
Dogs	42.4	56.3	937	640

Table II. Clinical laboratory studies related to the safety of ketoconazole

Patient population	Study design	Ketoconazole treatment			Safety investigations[1]	
		daily dose (mg)	duration of therapy	no. of subjects	type	frequency
Patients with superficial and/or deep mycoses	Open	200 (100-800)	97.5 days (4-428)	396 (782)[2]	Blood counts and chemistry	Prestudy, after about 1, 3, 6, 12 and 18 months of treatment
Patients with advanced malignancies, receiving cytostatics and immunotherapy	Open	200	1 year (3 months-1 year)	22	Blood counts and chemistry, visual acuity and slit-lamp examinations	Prestudy, after 1, 3, 6, and 12 months in study, and after study
Patients with onychomycosis	Controlled	200	9 months	123[3]	Blood counts and chemistry	Prestudy and after 3, 6 and 9 months in study
Patients with onychomycosis	Controlled	400	23 weeks	9[4]	Blood counts and chemistry	Prestudy and after 2, 4, 8, 16, 24 and 28 weeks of the study, and 4 weeks after treatment ended
		200	23 weeks	9		
Patients with vulvo-vaginitis	Open	600	3 days	13	Blood counts and chemistry	Prestudy, end of treatment, and 4 days after treatment
Patients with oral and/or intestinal mycoses	Open	400	2 weeks	30	Blood counts and chemistry	Prestudy and end of treatment
Patients with systemic or superficial mycoses	Open	200 (200-400)	145 days (8-377)	92	Slit-lamp eye examinations	Before and during treatment
Patient with hard palate and mandible lesions due to coccidioidomycosis	Open	200	7 months	1	Technetium pyro-phosphate bone scan	Before and after 4 and 7 months of treatment[5]
Patients with bone lesions due to coccidioidomycosis or North-American blastomycosis	Open	200-400	≥6 months	2	Bone x-rays	Before and during treatment
		200-400	≥3 months	2	Bone densitometry	Before and during treatment
Normal volunteers stabilised on warfarin	Open	200	21 days	2	Prothrombin time and ketoconazole metabolism	Every 2 days[6]

1 Based on unpublished data, on file Janssen Research Foundation, except where otherwise indicated.
2 Laboratory determinations in 782 patients, but detailed statistical analysis of data made on a sample of 396 patients.
3 A control group of 41 patients was followed during the same period.
4 A control group of 9 patients was followed during the same period.
5 Graybill et al. (in press).
6 Brass et al. (1979).

Oligodactylia and syndactylia occurred in most pups of female rats receiving food containing ketoconazole 80 and 160mg/kg. No abnormalities occurred at lower doses.

Mutagenicity and Carcinogenicity

In standard studies for mutagenicity, including the *in vitro* Ames test, the dominant lethal test in male and female mice, and the micronucleus test in mice, ketoconazole did not show mutagenic properties. Life-span oral carcinogenicity studies are at present underway in mice and rats.

Ophthalmic Toxicity

Topical application of 1% ketoconazole did not significantly retard the closure of corneal epithelial defects in rabbits, or produce other symptoms such as conjunctival injection, stromal oedema or iritis.

Safety Studies In Man

In a number of clinical studies laboratory investigations directed at monitoring biochemical effects of ketoconazole (table II) have been performed. No toxicity was observed related to the haematological system, the eye, liver or kidney function and electrolyte balance. Additionally, as a result of the tendency toward bone fragility seen in female rats during toxicity studies, a number of parameters related to bone formation were studied in man. No adverse changes in bone density or formation occurred in the small number of patients studied, and there were no abnormal elevations of serum calcium or alkaline phosphatase or decreases in serum phosphorus. Indeed, in a few patients with bone lesions due to fungal infections new bone formation occurred during treatment.

References

Brass, C.; Galgiani, J.N. and Stevens, D.A.: Treatment of coccidioidomycosis with oral ketoconazole. Proceedings of the 24th Annual Coccidioidomycosis Study Group Meeting, Las Vegas, Nevada, May 15 (1979).

Graybill, J.R.; Herndon, J.H.; Kniker, W.T. and Levine, H.B.: Ketoconazole treatment of chronic mucocutaneous candidiasis. Archives of Dermatology 116: 1137-1147 (1980).

Ketoconazole: Clinical Experience in Superficial Mycoses

A new drug for oral administration in the treatment of superficial mycoses must be of considerable interest to all involved in the therapy of such conditions. Orally administered ketoconazole has been studied in a variety of the more common superficial fungal infections. As shown in table I (and as is discussed in more detail in chapters VIII to XIII which follow) results have been most encouraging. Although in some areas further data must accumulate before definitive statements on the relative efficacy of ketoconazole can be made, it seems that the drug represents a step forward in the treatment of superficial fungal disease.

Table I. Summary of the effectiveness of orally administered ketoconazole in various superficial mycoses

Condition (number of patients)[1]	Response (%)		
	remission	remission or marked improvement	overall efficacy[2]
Dermatomycoses (454)	67	88	+ + +
Tinea capitis and favus (43)	28	58	+ +(?)
Pityriasis versicolor (223)	92	98	+ + +
Oral thrush (57)	77	84	+ + +
Vaginal candidosis (826)	75-90[3]		+ + +
Chronic mucocutaneous candidosis (69)	25	77	+ + +
Onychomycoses (115)	68	81	+ + +

1 Multicentre patients.
2 + + + = highly effective; + + = moderately effective (based on response in the multicentre study and subsequent published and unpublished evidence).
3 Response with various dosage schedules involving a total dose of $\geqslant$ 1200mg.

Chapter VIII

Dermatomycoses
(figs. 1 to 5)

Superficial infections caused by dermatophytes or yeasts are the most common form of fungal disease. A wide variety of topical agents has been used in their treatment. Topical therapy, in particular with those agents developed in recent years, is usually effective in such conditions if an adequate course of therapy is completed, but this mode of treatment may be an inconvenience to some patients, and may be less effective if hairy areas of the body are involved. Griseofulvin is effective in most skin and scalp infections due to dermatophytes, but it is not effective in yeast infections.

More than 500 patients with dermatophyte or yeast infections of the skin, including 42 children with scalp infections, have been treated with orally administered ketoconazole (Botter et al., 1979: Drouhet and Dupont, 1980; Haneke, 1981; Jones et al., 1981; Legendre and Steltz, 1980; Robertson et al., 1980; Vladez and Tuculet, 1979; Welsh and Rodriguez, 1980; unpublished data on file, Janssen Research Foundation).

Open Studies in Skin Infections

Study Methods

In a large multicentre study 483 patients with fungal skin infections were treated by 67 investigators. Infecting fungi were demonstrated by microscopic and/or culture methods in all patients. *Trichophyton rubrum*, *Trichophyton mentagrophytes*, *Epidermophyton floccosum*, *Microsporum canis*, *Candida albicans* and *Candida tropicalis* were the organisms most frequently encountered. The median duration of the fungal infection was 4 months (range of 7 days to 49 years).

187 patients had failed to respond to or had relapsed after previous antifungal treatment; previous therapy included a wide variety of topical antifungal agents, as well as systemic therapy with griseofulvin or in a few patients amphotericin B, econazole or miconazole.

The dosage of ketoconazole was usually 200mg once daily taken with a meal, for a median of 4 weeks prior to evaluation (range of 1 to 38 weeks). Evaluation was based on both clinical and mycological response.

Results

Remission occurred in 67% of 454 cases, marked improvement in 21%, moderate improvement in 10% with no change in 2% (table I). Interestingly, 3 patients with *T. rubrum* infections shown to be griseofulvin-resistant *in vitro* responded well to ketoconazole therapy (Robertson et al., 1980). The median time to response (remission or marked improvement)

Table I. Results of the treatment of 454 cases of dermatophyte or yeast skin infections with orally administered ketoconazole

Clinical results	No. of patients (%)	Mycological evidence			Overall results[1]			
		negative	positive	not done	±	+	+ +	+ + +
No change	11 (2)	7	4					
Moderate improvement	47 (10)	29	12	6				
Marked improvement	83 (18)	29	16	38				
Clinical cure	275 (61)	11	104	160				
Not evaluable	38 (8)			38				
All cases	454 (100)	76 (17)	136 (30)	242 (53)	11 (2)	47 (10)	94 (21)	302 (67)

1   ± = no change, + = moderate improvement, + + = marked improvement, + + + = remission.

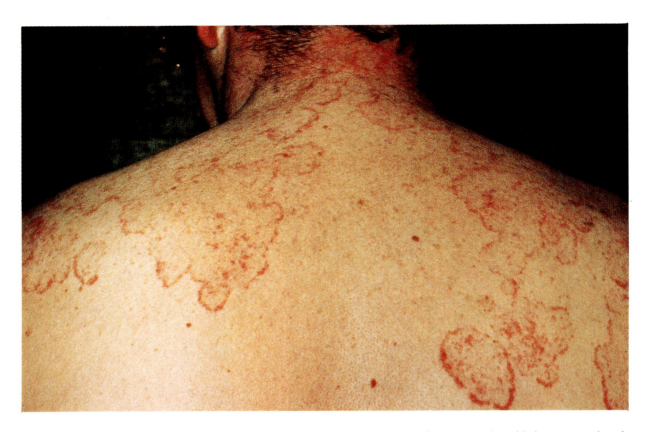

Fig. 1. A patient with tinea corporis *(Trichophyton rubrum)* before and after treatment with ketoconazole administered orally for 1 month. (By courtesy of Professor Dr H. Grimmer, Chef Arzt der Dermatologischer Klinik, Wiesbaden)

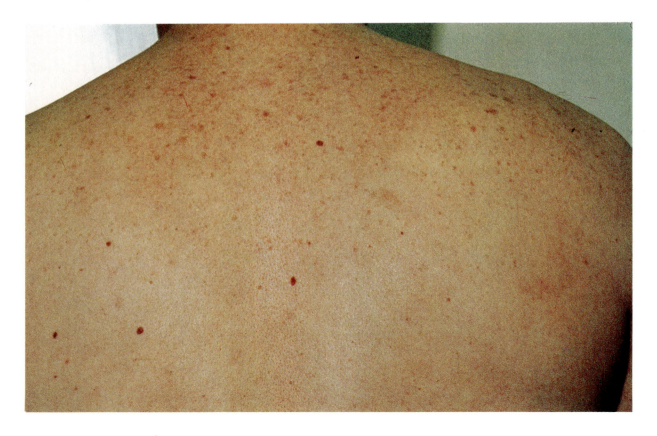

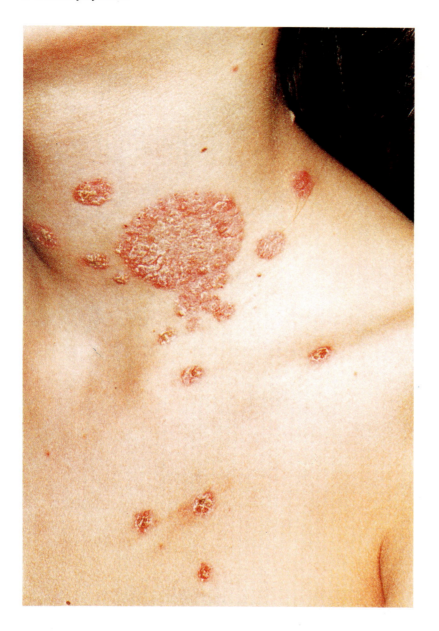

Fig. 2. A patient with tinea corporis *(Trichophyton verrucosum)* before and after treatment with orally administered ketoconazole for 1 month. (By courtesy of Dr A. Englehardt, Hautfacharzt Stationäre Behandlung Hautklinik, Rottweil, Germany)

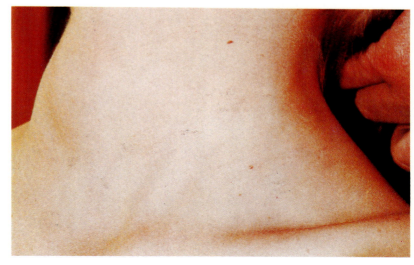

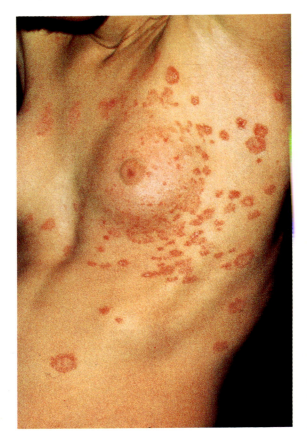

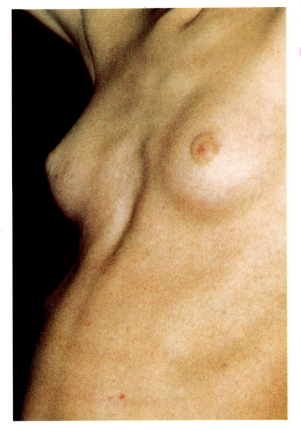

Fig. 3. A patient with tinea corporis (organism not identified) before and after treatment with orally administered ketoconazole for 1 month. (By courtesy of Dr A. Englehardt, Hautfacharzt Stationäre Behandlung Hautklinik, Rottweil, Germany)

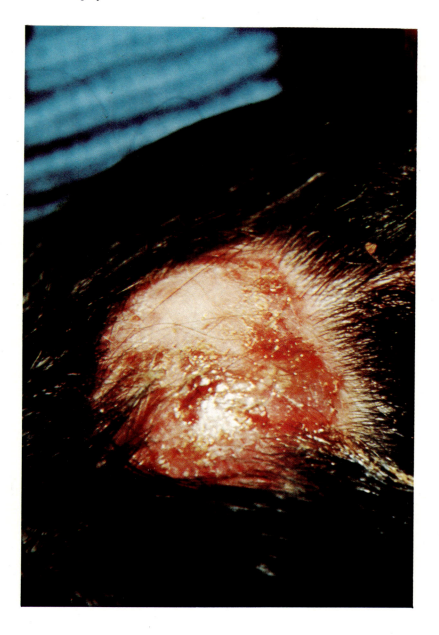

Fig. 4. A patient with tinea capitis before and after treatment with orally administered ketoconazole for 3 weeks. (Courtesy Dr R. Galimberti, Hospital Italiano, Buenos Aires)

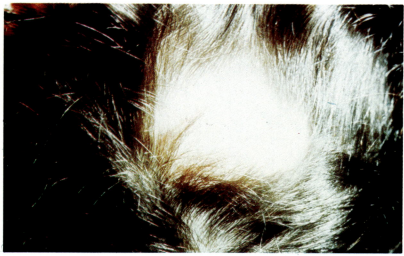

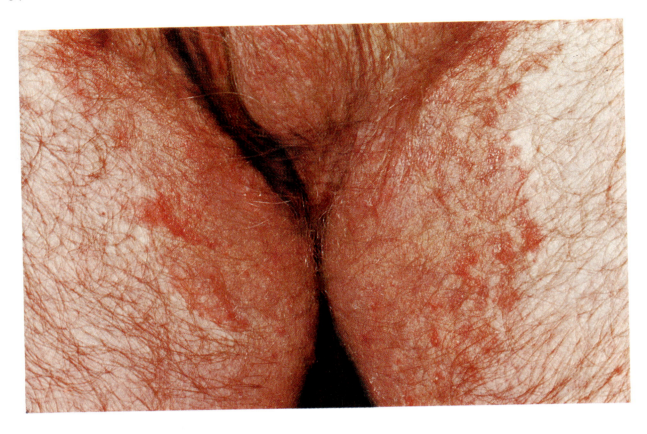

Fig. 5. A patient with tinea cruris *(Trichophyton rubrum)* before and after treatment with ketoconazole orally for 4 months. (By courtesy of Dr A. Englehardt, Hautfacharzt Stationäre Behandlung Hautklinik, Rottweil, Germany)

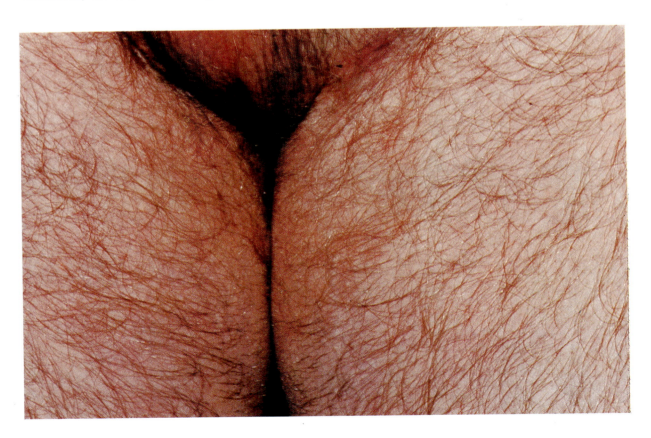

was 4 weeks (fig. 6). Yeast infections tended to respond slightly more rapidly than dermatophyte infections, particularly those due to *T. rubrum*.

On clinical assessment, lesions on the trunk cleared most rapidly, followed by those on the hands and lastly those on the feet (Robertson et al., 1980). In *dermatophyte infections* symptoms such as inflammation, exudation, erythema, vesicles and fissures cleared rapidly, but as might be expected desquamation was slower to respond (fig. 7). The time course of symptomatic improvement in *yeast infections* was not evaluated in most patients.

Open Studies in Scalp Infections

Study Methods

39 children (aged 1 to 15 years) with tinea capitis and three with favus were treated with ketoconazole in a multicentre study involving 12 investigators. A single adult with tinea capitis caused by *M. canis*, and unresponsive to griseofulvin, has also been treated successfully (Van Hecke and Meysman, 1980).

In the multicentre study *M. canis* was demonstrated in 17 children, *Microsporum audouini* in 1 child, *Trichophyton violaceum* in 9 children, *Trichophyton tonsurans* in 8, *Trichophyton schoenleini* in 3, *Trichophyton soudanense* in 2, and *Trichophyton mentagrophytes* and *verrucosum* in 1 each. Most patients had not received previous antifungal treatment.

Ketoconazole was administered orally in a median dose of 6.25mg/kg daily (range of 3.5 to 13mg/kg/day). Evaluation based on clinical and mycological response took place after a median of 5 weeks of treatment (range of 2 to 39 weeks).

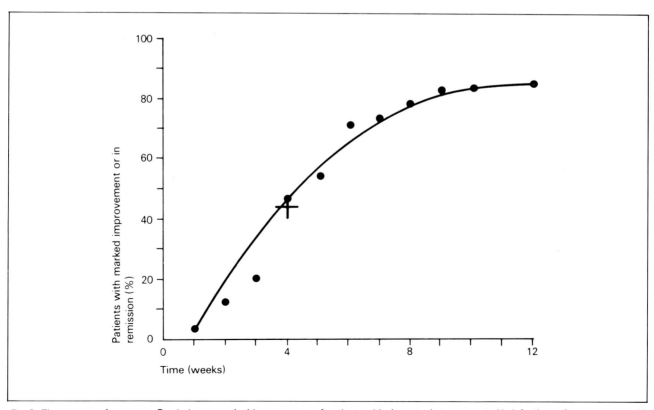

Fig. 6. Time course of response. Remission or marked improvement of patients with dermatophyte or yeast skin infections after treatment with orally administered ketoconazole. The cross indicates the median.

Results

Remission occurred in 28% of cases, marked improvement in 30%, moderate improvement in 28% and no change was seen in 14% (table II). The median time to response was 4 weeks.

In tinea capitis results were significantly better (p = 0.01) when the fungus involved was of the 'human type' (species of *Trichophyton, M. audouini*) than when fungi from animal sources (*M. canis*) were involved, possibly related to an inadequate duration of treatment in patients with *M. canis* infections (usually only 1-2 months). Nevertheless, several patients with *M. canis* infections showed moderate improvement and a few achieved marked improvement or remission. Thus, comparative response rates were 73% of infections involving species of *Trichophyton* versus 29% of *M. canis* infections. The 3 patients with favus (*T. schoenleini*) were markedly improved at the time of evaluation.

Controlled Studies

In a double-blind comparative study in the USA, in patients with fungal skin infections usually due to species of *Trichophyton*, ketoconazole 200mg daily was clearly more effective than griseofulvin 250mg daily (ultramicrosize preparation, Fulvicin P/G®-Schering USA), each given for 2 to 16 weeks prior to evaluation (Legendre and Steltz, 1980; unpublished data, on file Janssen Research Foundation). 61% of 66 ketoconazole-treated patients and 39% of 64 griseofulvin-treated patients

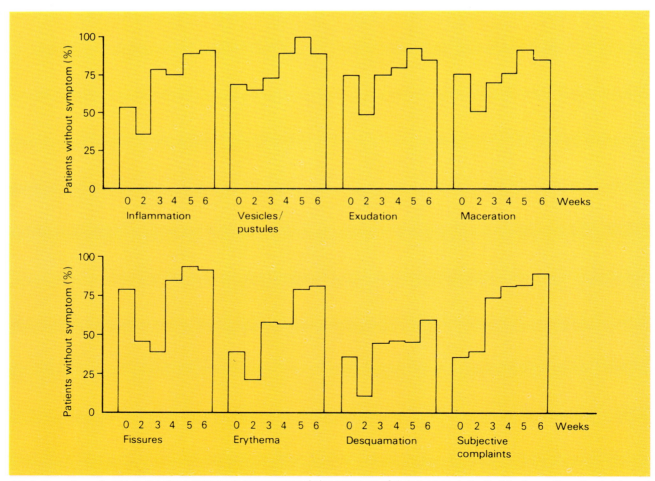

Fig. 7. Percentage of patients showing symptomatic improvement during treatment of their dermatophyte skin infections with orally administered ketoconazole. (Not all patients were evaluated at 2 weeks.)

Table II. Results of treatment of 43 cases (42 patients) of tinea capitis or favus (3 patients) with orally administered ketoconazole

Clinical results	No. of patients (%)	Mycological evidence			Overall results[1]			
		negative	positive	not done	±	+	+ +	+ + +
No change	6 (14)		5	1				
Moderate improvement	12 (28)		12					
Marked improvement	12 (28)	6	5	1				
Clinical cure	12 (28)	9	1	2				
Not evaluable	1 (2)	1						
All cases	43 (100)	16 (37)	23 (53)	4 (9)	6 (14)	12 (28)	13 (30)	12 (28)

1 ± = no change; + = moderate improvement; + + = marked improvement; + + + = remission.

achieved remission, and relapse occurred less frequently in patients who had received ketoconazole (table III). Similarly, in comparative studies conducted outside the USA, 71 % of 73 patients resonded to ketoconazole (200mg daily) at 4 weeks, and 86 % at the end of treatment, compared with 40 % and 71 %, respectively, in those receiving griseofulvin 500mg daily (microsize).

In the comparative studies above 18 patients with *T. tonsurans* achieved remission or marked improvement, after a median of 4 weeks, in 8 of 10 ketoconazole-treated and 6 of 8 griseofulvin-treated patients.

Factors Affecting Response

Fungal Skin Infections

As mentioned above, yeast infections tended to respond slightly more rapidly than dermatophyte infections, but the ultimate response rates were similar in both groups. Lesions on the hands or feet or generalised skin lesions responded more slowly to ketoconazole therapy (about a 55 to 60 % decrease in the number of lesions at the time of evaluation) than those in other specific areas of the body (about a 70 to 100 % decrease in the number of lesions).

Other variables such as the dose of ketoconazole, previous antifungal treatment, sex, immunodeficiency, diabetes mellitus, thyroid dysfunction, neoplasms, renal failure or concurrent antibiotic therapy did not influence the response to ketoconazole.

Relapse

Fungal Skin Infections

In the open studies, of 64 patients in remission who discontinued treatment and were followed for up to 3 months, 56 % relapsed in the first month after treatment, 13 % in the second month and 3 % in the third month. 18 patients (28 %) were still in remission 3 months after ending

Table III. Comparative effectiveness of griseofulvin and ketoconazole in patients with fungal skin infections (see also text for results in additional comparative studies)

Efficacy	Griseofulvin-treated patients (n = 64)	Ketoconazole-treated patients (n = 66)
Remission	39 %	61 %
Marked improvement	36 %	27 %
Moderate improvement or no change	25 %	12 %
Relapse rate[1]	10/23 (43 %)	3/35 (9 %)

1 Follow-up duration 4 months.

treatment. In contrast, a much smaller proportion of ketoconazole-treated patients relapsed (3 of 35 = 9%) in a 4-month follow-up period after a double-blind study (see table III). Whether the high incidence of early relapses is due to premature discontinuation of treatment will be an interesting area for further study.

Fungal Scalp Infections in Children

One of 12 children with tinea capitis who achieved remission during treatment with ketoconazole received continued therapy to prevent relapse. Four children in remission who discontinued treatment were followed-up for 1 month or less; 3 of them remained in remission while the fourth relapsed but subsequently achieved remission again following re-treatment with ketoconazole for 29 days.

Conclusions

In patients with fungal skin infections due to either dermatophytes or yeasts the response rate seen with orally administered ketoconazole therapy is most encouraging. In infections due to species of *Trichophyton* ketoconazole appears to be at least as effective as griseofulvin; in *M. canis* or *E. floccosum* infections the relative effectiveness of the two drugs is less clearly established.

The results achieved in children with tinea capitis are also of considerable interest, particularly since the median time to response was a relatively short period of 4 weeks. However, infections of the scalp due to fungi from animal sources (*M. canis*) took longer to heal than *Trichophyton* infections; the role of ketoconazole in treating tinea capitis due to the former requires additional study.

In both skin and scalp infections further follow-up data are needed to clarify the likelihood of relapse after achieving remission with ketoconazole therapy.

In summary, with activity against both dermatophyte and yeast infections, ketoconazole is the first orally absorbed broad spectrum antifungal drug for treating superficial skin infections, and must thus be regarded as an important advance in therapy.

References

Botter, A.A.; Dethier, F.; Mertens, R.L.J.; Morias, J. and Peremans, W.: Skin and nail mycoses: treatment with ketoconazole, a new oral antimycotic agent. Mykosen 22: 274-278 (1979).

Drouhet, E. and Dupont, B.: Chronic mucocutaneous candidosis and other superficial and systemic mycoses successfully treated with ketoconazole. Reviews of Infectious Diseases 2: 606-619 (1980).

Haneke, E.: Ketoconazole treatment of dermatomycoses. International Congress of Chemotherapy, Florence, Italy, 19-24 July (1981).

Jones, H.E.; Simpson, J.G. and Artis, W.M.: Oral ketoconazole: an effective and safe treatment for dermatophytosis. Archives of Dermatology 117: 129-134 (1981).

Legendre, R. and Steltz, M.: A multi-center, double-blind comparison of ketoconazole and griseofulvin in the treatment of infections due to dermatophytes. Reviews of Infectious Diseases 2: 586-591 (1980).

Robertson, M.H.; Hanifin, J.M. and Parker, F.: Oral therapy with ketoconazole for dermatophyte infections unresponsive to griseofulvin. Reviews of Infectious Diseases 2: 578-581 (1980).

Valdez, R. and Tuculet, M.A.: Dermatomicosis extensa en una paciente sometida a corticoterapia. Revista Argentina de Micologia 2: 27-29 (1979).

Van Hecke, E. and Meysman, L.: Tinea capitis in an adult (*Microsporum canis*). Mykosen 23: 607-608 (1980).

Welsh, O. and Rodriguez, M.: Treatment of dermatomycoses with ketoconazole. Reviews of Infectious Diseases 2: 582-585 (1980).

Chapter IX

Pityriasis Versicolor
(fig. 1)

Pityriasis versicolor (tinea versicolor) is caused by a superficial skin infection with *Malassezia furfur (Pityrosporum orbiculare)*. It is characterised by brown, red or at times achromatic scaly patches which occur principally on the trunk but which may be found anywhere on the skin. Traditionally it has been treated with topical antifungal agents (Conant et al., 1971; Ive, 1973).

About 300 patients with pityriasis versicolor have been treated with orally administered ketoconazole (Borelli, 1980; Borelli et al., 1979a,b,; del Palacio Hernanz et al., 1980; Jolliffe and Ngai, in manuscript; Welsh and Rodriguez, 1980; unpublished data, on file Janssen Research Foundation).

Open Studies

Study Methods

In a multicentre study 223 patients were treated by 43 investigators. *Malassezia furfur* was demonstrated by microscopy in most patients and confirmed under Wood's light examination in some. *Pityrosporum ovale* was cultured in 8 patients. 83 patients had failed to respond to or had relapsed after their last antifungal treatment, which included topical econazole, miconazole, clotrimazole, nystatin, tolnaftate, other topical agents or, in a few patients, griseofulvin. 106 patients had not received previous antifungal treatment.

Most patients received a single daily dose of 200mg of ketoconazole administered with a meal, for a period of 1 to 15 weeks (median 4 weeks). Evaluation was based on clinical and mycological responses, and in 59 patients on symptomatic relief also.

Response to Ketoconazole

Overall results of treatment with ketoconazole in 223 patients showed a remission rate of 92.4% (206 patients), with marked improvement in 5.4% (12 patients), moderate improvement in 1.8% (4 patients) and no change in a single patient (table I). The median time for response (remission or marked improvement) was about 3 weeks (fig. 2).

Table I. Results of the treatment of 223 patients with pityriasis versicolor with orally administered ketoconazole

Clinical results	No. of patients (%)	Mycological evidence			Overall results[1]			
		negative	positive	not done	±	+	+ +	+ + +
No change	1 (0.4)		1					
Moderate improvement	4 (1.8)	1	2	1				
Marked improvement	11 (5)	3	3	5				
Clinical cure	194 (87)	97	1	96				
Not evaluable	13 (5.8)	13	0	0				
All patients	223 (100)	114 (51)	7 (3)	102 (46)	1 (0.4)	4 (1.8)	12 (5.4)	206 (92.4)

1 ± = no change; + = moderate improvement; + + = marked improvement; + + + = remission.

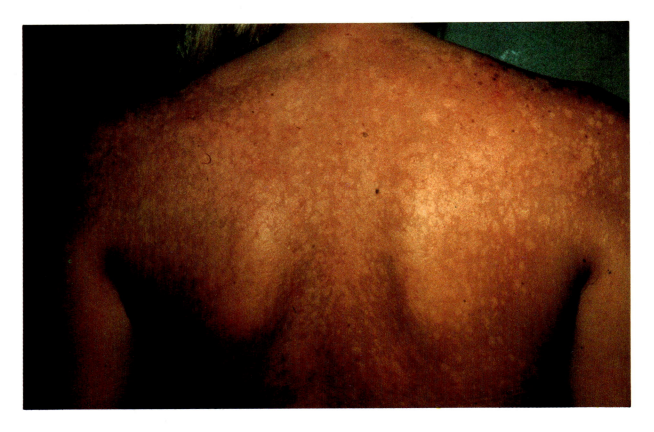

Fig. 1. Response of patient with pityriasis versicolor to oral treatment with ketoconazole. Before and after treatment for 1 month. (By courtesy of Dr R. Galimberti, Hospital Italiano, Buenos Aires).

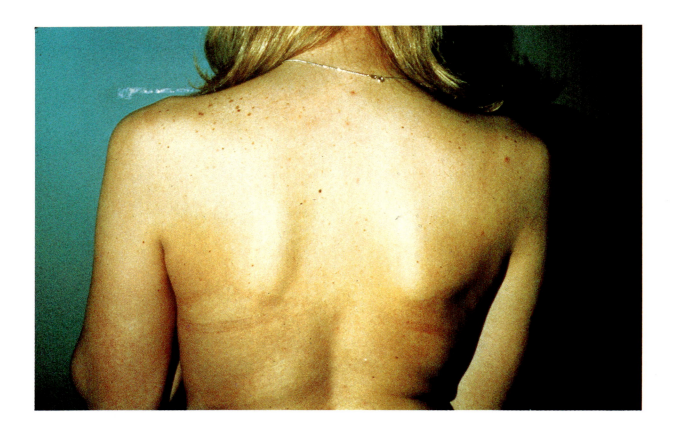

Some symptomatic improvement occurred rapidly, with most patients free of erythema and inflammation within 2 to 3 weeks, although desquamation was slightly less amenable to therapy (fig. 3), and residual hypopigmented macules often persisted for up to 6 months after treatment ended (Borelli, 1980).

Controlled Studies

In a double-blind placebo controlled study, using similar criteria for diagnosis and evaluation as the open studies described above (*Malassezia furfur* demonstrated by microscopy and confirmed under Wood's light in all patients), 20 patients with pityriasis versicolor were randomly assigned to treatment with either ketoconazole 200mg daily or placebo for 2 weeks. Remission or marked improvement occurred in 9 of 10 ketoconazole-treated patients and 2 of 10 control patients, when evaluated 2 weeks after the end of treatment, and in 7 of 10 and 1 of 10 patients receiving ketoconazole and placebo, respectively, when evaluated immediately after the 2-week treatment period.

Factors Affecting Response

Although most patients received a dose of 200mg once daily for several weeks, a small number of patients received higher (400mg daily) or lower (as little as 200mg once weekly) doses, or a single dose of 400mg (Borelli, 1980). No clear dose-response relationship has been established. Several patients were considered 'cured' after single doses.

Neither the extent of lesions nor the duration of the disease correlated with the response rate. Results were also similar in patients who had received previous antifungal therapy and in those being treated for the first time.

Relapse

In one series, re-infection occurred in 6 of 78 patients considered 'cured' (Borelli, 1980); most of these had received low dose or single dose therapy (see above). In 2 of these re-infected patients lesions were more numerous than previously. Re-infected patients responded readily to subsequent treatment with ketoconazole, often to a single dose of 400mg.

A small number of patients received ketoconazole prophylactically in a dose of 200mg monthly to prevent relapse, but further experience is needed before the effectiveness of such therapy can be stated with any certainty.

Conclusions

Orally administered ketoconazole is an effective treatment for pityriasis versicolor. A dose of 200mg once daily produces rapid improvement, with most patients in remission or markedly improved in 4 to 6 weeks or less.

Some areas remain to be further clarified, including optimum dosage schedule and duration of treatment; there is some early evidence that a single dose, or intermittent administration every few days, or even weekly, may be effective. The possibility of an effective single dose regimen is certainly exciting, and should be thoroughly investigated. Assuming that ketoconazole reaches the superficial site of infection as a result of excretion with sebum (see chapter 6), the effect of bathing on the outcome of therapy needs to be investigated. Is frequent bathing likely to augment

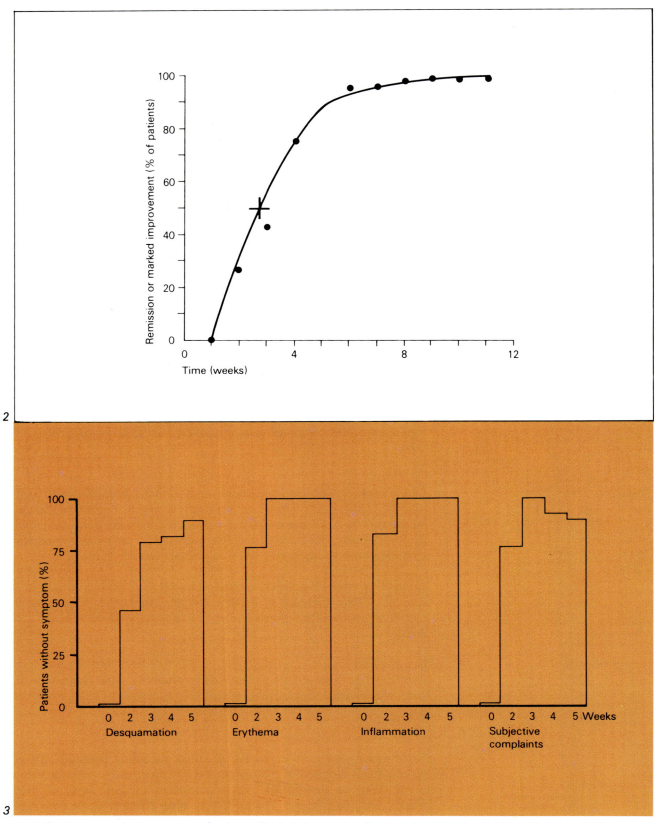

Fig. 2. Remission or marked improvement of patients with pityriasis versicolor after treatment with orally administered ketoconazole. The cross indicates the median.

Fig. 3. Percentage of patients with pityriasis versicolor who were free of symptoms after 2, 3, 4 and 5 weeks treatment with orally administered ketoconazole.

the response as a result of improved hygiene, or to reduce the response by removing the drug from the skin, or neither? Such a consideration could be of particular importance if single dose or intermittent dose treatment regimens prove to be effective.

Re-infection is a common problem in patients with pityriasis versicolor, and the effectiveness of prophylactic regimens of ketoconazole to prevent relapse needs to be carefully examined.

References

Borelli, D.: Treatment of pityriasis versicolor with ketoconazole. Reviews of Infectious Diseases 2: 592-595 (1980).

Borelli, D.; Fuentes, J.; Leiderman, E.; Restrepo-M.A.; Bran, J.L.; Legendre, R.; Levine, H.B. and Stevens, D.A.: Ketoconazole, an oral antifungal: laboratory and clinical assessment of imidazole drugs. Postgraduate Medical Journal 55: 657-661 (1979a).

Borelli, D.; Marcano, R. and Marcano, C.: Pitiriasis versicolor: tratamiento per os con ketoconazole. Revista Fundacion J.M. Vargas 3: 19-23 (1979b).

Conant, N.F.; Smith, D.T.; Baker, R.D. and Callaway, J.L.: Manual of Clinical Mycology, p.644-651 (Saunders, Philadelphia 1971).

Ive, F.A.: Diseases of the skin. Treatment of skin infections and infestations. British Medical Journal 4: 475-478 (1973).

del Palacio Hernanz, A.; Herino Luque, V.; Iglesias Diez, L.; Barlett Coma, A. and Sanz Sanz, F.: Ensayo clinico con ketoconazol en pitiriasis versicolor. 2nd Symposium de Dermatologistes de la Securite Sociale, Madrid (1980).

Welsh, O. and Rodriguez, M.: Treatment of dermatomycoses with ketoconazole. Reviews of Infectious Diseases 2: 582-585 (1980).

Chapter X

Oral Candidosis
(Thrush)
(fig. 1)

Candida albicans is a normal inhabitant of the oral cavity, but in certain conditions a state of overgrowth develops with resulting oral infection, accompanied in some patients by gastrointestinal or vaginal infection. Candidal overgrowth is most likely to occur at the extremes of age, or in debilitated patients, and in those receiving prolonged therapy with corticosteroids, immunosuppressives or broad spectrum antibiotics (Zegarelli, 1980).

A relatively small number of adult patients (56) with oral thrush have been treated with orally administered ketoconazole in a multicentre study (Borelli et al., 1979; unpublished data, on file Janssen Research Foundation). 50 children ranging from 2 weeks to 30 months of age have also been treated, using a suspension dosage form (Cauwenbergh et al., 1981).

Open Studies

Study Methods

Candida was demonstrated by culture in all patients in the multicentre study, excepting one individual in whom direct microscopic examination was positive. *Candida* spp. was cultured in 40 patients, *Candida albicans* in 13, *Candida parapsilosis* in 1 and *Candida krusei* in 1. The median duration of the presenting episode of thrush was 1 week, but ranged up to 5 years. 45 patients had not received previous treatment with antifungal drugs, while 9 patients had failed to respond adequately to previous treatment with intravenous amphotericin B, topical miconazole, oral or topical nystatin, or natamycin. Treatment with ketoconazole usually consisted of 1 or 2 tablets (200mg per tablet) daily, taken with a meal.

Response to Ketoconazole

Remission occurred in 77 % of patients (44 of 57 treatment courses, 1 patient receiving a second course of treatment following a relapse), and marked or moderate improvement in 7 % each (4 of 57 patients, each). No change was seen in 9 % (5 cases) [table I]. The median time to response was 1 week, with most responses occurring within 3 weeks or less (fig. 2).

In 50 children (infants to 30 months of age) with clinically evident thrush, administration of ketoconazole in a suspension formulation (20mg/ml, 1ml given 3 times daily for up to 2 weeks) was highly effective (Cauwenbergh et al., 1981; unpublished data, on file Janssen Research Foundation). Marked symptomatic improvement occurred in 96 % of patients, and the incidence of positive cultures was reduced to 19 % compared with

Table I. Results of ketoconazole treatment in 56 adult patients (57 treatment courses) with oral candidosis (see also text for data in children)

Clinical result	No. of patients (%)	Mycological evidence			Overall results[1]			
		negative	positive	not done	±	+	+ +	+ + +
No change	5 (9)		4	1				
Moderate improvement	4 (7)	1	2	1				
Marked improvement	3 (5)		3					
Clinical cure	42 (74)	36	1	5				
Not evaluable	3 (5)	3						
All patients	57 (100)	40 (70)	10 (18)	7 (12)	5 (9)	4 (7)	4 (7)	44 (77)

1 ± = no change; + = moderate improvement; + + = marked improvement; + + + = remission.

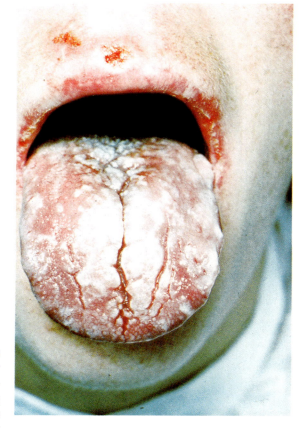

Fig. 1. Patient with chronic oral thrush before and after treatment with orally administered ketoconazole (200mg once daily) for 1 week. (See also chapter XII). [By courtesy of Dr R.J. Hay, London School of Hygiene and Tropical Medicine, and the Department of Medical Photography, St. John's Hospital for Diseases of the Skin]

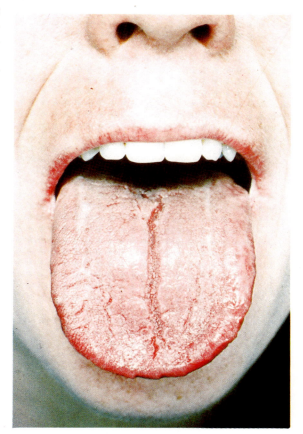

94% before treatment. Of 26 children with symptoms thought to be related to gastrointestinal candidosis, 12 still had symptoms after 1 week's treatment with ketoconazole and only 4 after 2 weeks' treatment. Diaper rash disappeared in all 14 patients with this symptom after 2 weeks' treatment.

Factors Affecting Response

The response rate was not related to the duration of the presenting episode of candidosis, nor to the dosage of ketoconazole (fig. 3). There was no difference in response between previously untreated patients and those who had not responded adequately to previous antifungal agents.

A small number of patients with immunodeficiencies or diabetes mellitus tended to respond less readily than the group as a whole (fig. 4). The

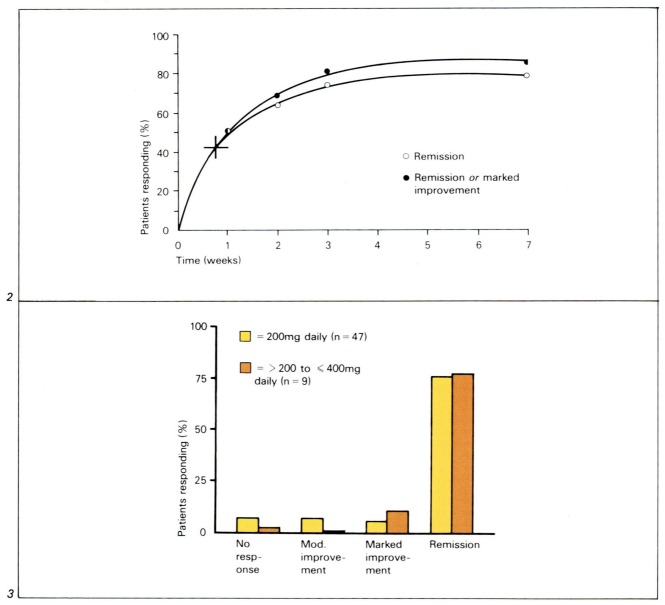

Response of oral candidosis to ketoconazole.

Fig. 2. Time course of response of 56 patients (57 treatment courses). The cross indicates the median.

Fig. 3. Response in patients receiving different doses of ketoconazole.

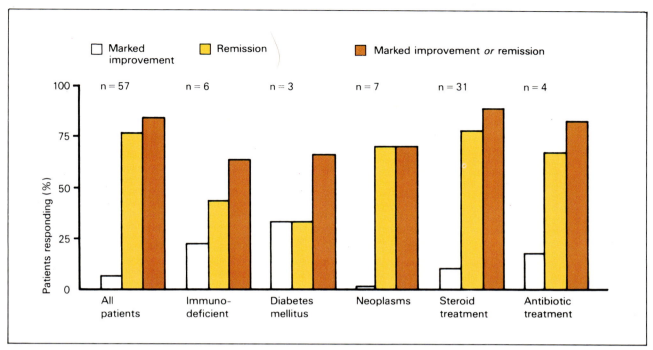

Fig. 4. The effect of predisposing conditions or concomitant disease in patients with oral candidosis treated with ketoconazole.

response in patients with neoplasms, and those receiving corticosteroids or antibiotics was similar to that of the entire group.

Relapse

The relapse rate following successful treatment of oral candidosis with ketoconazole has not been well documented as yet. A single patient followed for 4 months after treatment remained in remission. Another patient who discontinued treatment after 3 weeks, when he was clinically free of symptoms but still had positive cultures, relapsed in the second month of follow-up. A few patients have received prophylactic ketoconazole therapy to prevent relapse.

Conclusions

Orally administered ketoconazole produces rapid remission in about 75 to 80% of adults and 96% of children with oral candidosis, although the response may be lower in patients with certain predisposing factors. A dose of 200mg daily is as effective as a higher dose in adults and the effective dose in children is 1mg 3 times a day. Further studies are needed to define the relapse rate after successful treatment, and to establish more clearly the role of prophylactic ketoconazole administration in 'at risk' patients.

References

Borelli, D.; Juentes, J.; Leiderman, E.; Restrepo-M., A.; Bran, J.L.; Legendre, R.; Levine, H.B. and Stevens, D.A.: Ketoconazole, an oral antifungal: Laboratory and clinical assessment of imidazole drugs. Postgraduate Medical Journal 55: 657-661 (1979).

Cauwenbergh, G.; Casneuf, J.; de Loore, F.; Poot, J.; Van den Bon, P. and Vay Eygen, M.: Treatment of infant thrush with ketoconazole, a new orally absorbed broad spectrum antimycotic. International Congress of Chemotherapy, Florence, Italy, 19-24 July (1981).

Zegarelli, E.: Diseases of the oral cavity; in Avery (Ed) Drug Treatment, 2nd Edition, p.393-411 (Churchill Livingstone, Edinburgh and Adis Press, Sydney 1980).

Chapter XI

Vaginal Candidosis

Candida albicans is often present in the female genital tract without producing symptoms of infection. Clinical infection may occur in the presence of certain host factors, such as pregnancy, diabetes or immunodeficiency or local factors, such as altered pH whether hormonal contraception predisposes to infection is debatable (p.4). Treatment has traditionally consisted of the use of an effective anticandidal drug applied intravaginally; some advocate combination with an oral anticandidal agent to prevent reinfection from the bowel (Platts, 1980). That the treatment of this common condition needs further improvement is attested to by the large number of topical preparations available and the variation in length of the treatment courses recommended (Willcox, 1977).

Treatment of vaginal candidosis with orally administered ketoconazole has been studied in more than 800 patients (Bisschop et al., 1979; Creatsas et al., 1980; Fregosa-Duenas, 1980; del Palacio Hernanz et al., 1980; unpublished data, on file Janssen Research Foundation).

Open Studies

Study Methods

Most open studies have been conducted with protocols similar to that in a large multicentre study involving 498 patients. In this study all patients had clinically apparent vaginal candidosis, which was confirmed by microscopic and/or culture methods. *Candida albicans* was present in 492 patients, *Candida zeylonoides* in 1 patient. 18 patients had mixed infections of *Torulopsis glabrata* and *Candida* spp. and 2 patients had mixed *Candida* infections. In all studies patients were examined before and at 3 to 10 days after treatment, and in most studies again at 3 to 4 weeks after treatment. Evaluation was made on the basis of symptom scores and mycological results.

Various dosage schedules of ketoconazole were studied (see below).

Table I. Mycological results with various dosage schedules of orally administered ketoconazole in patients with vaginal candidosis (combined results of all available data)

Dosage schedule	Number of patients	Patients with negative culture (%)	
		at 3-10 days post-treatment	at 3-4 weeks post-treatment
100mg bid × 3 days	9	44	
100mg tid × 3 days	12	84	67
150mg tid × 3 days	16	75	44
200mg once daily × 3 days	212	68	61
200mg once daily × 6 days	34	82	76
200mg bid × 3 days	165	87	84
200mg bid × 6 days	39	90	83
200mg tid × 1 day	8	75	
200mg tid × 3 days	151	91	72
400mg once daily × 5 days	121	83	81
600mg single dose	27	59	
600mg once daily × 3 days	32	78	

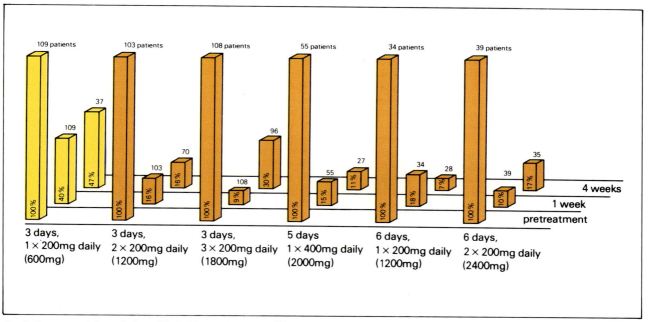

Fig. 1. Ketoconazole in vaginal candidosis. Mycological results (% of patients with positive cultures before and 1 week and 4 weeks after treatment) with various oral dosage schedules of ketoconazole in patients with vaginal candidoses. (Results of a multicentre study).

Results

The mycological results achieved with various dosage schedules are shown in table I and figure 1. Generally, dosage schedules involving a total dose of 1200mg or more produced negative cultures in at least 80% of patients. A dose of 200mg once daily for 6 days or twice daily for 3 days seemed most suitable, as little further improvement occurred with higher doses. A standard regimen of 200mg twice daily for 5 days is now advocated.

Symptomatic improvement occurred rapidly with dosage schedules of 1200mg total dose or more; vaginitis, vulvitis, pruritus vulvae and leucor-rhoea were markedly improved or absent in most patients with mycological cures (fig. 2), although leucorrhoea persisted in some patients.

Controlled Studies

In 2 double-blind studies in patients with vaginal candidosis comparing orally administered ketoconazole (200mg 3 times daily for 3 days) with miconazole administered intravaginally as a soft gelatin capsule in a relatively high dose/short term schedule (400mg 3 times daily for 3 days), both drugs were highly effective when evaluated shortly after treatment ended (table II). However, mycological relapse occurred more frequently in ketoconazole-treated patients (see table). In one such study, of 7 patients who relapsed after ketoconazole therapy and were subsequently treated and 'cured' with topical miconazole, relapse again occurred in 5 patients after 28 days, suggesting that these patients were particularly prone to re-infection.

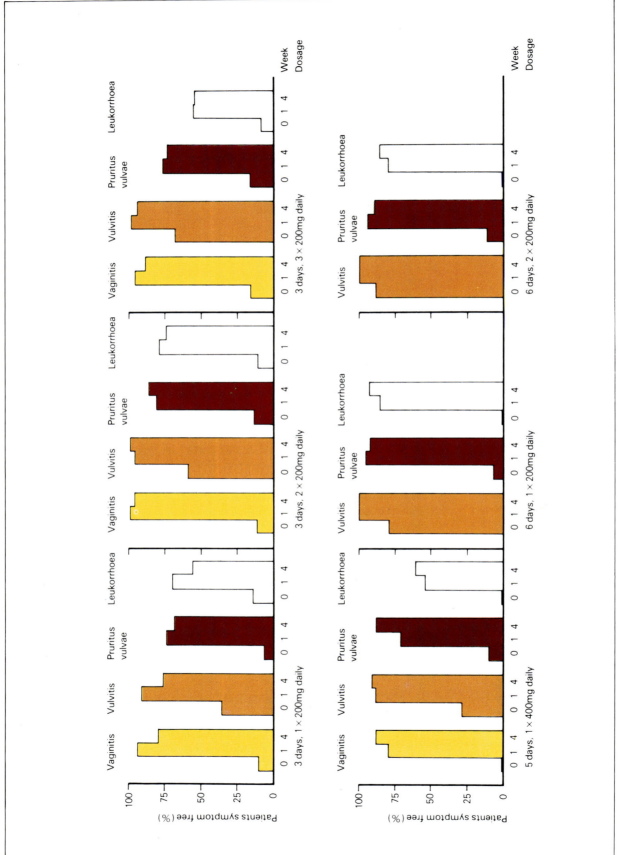

Fig. 2. Symptomatic improvement in 498 patients with vaginal candidosis treated orally with ketoconazole in various dosage schedules.

Factors Affecting Response

Provided at least a total of 1200mg of ketoconazole is administered, the dosage schedule chosen appears to have little influence on the mycological outcome of therapy. The influence of other factors such as hormonal contraceptives, diabetes mellitus, immunodeficiency or treatment of the sexual partner(s) on the response rate cannot be determined from the available data.

Relapse

When patients were followed-up for 4 weeks after treatment with ketoconazole the incidence of relapse varied from 7 to 30% with a total administered dose of at least 1200mg (see fig. 1). In double-blind studies the incidence of mycological relapse with ketoconazole was greater than with miconazole given intravaginally, but this may have been due to a preponderance of 'relapse prone' patients in the ketoconazole group in one study.

Conclusions

Orally administered ketoconazole is clearly an effective treatment for vaginal candidosis. The availability of an effective agent for oral therapy of this common condition, which has previously required local therapy with all the attendant problems of inconvenience to the patient and the resultant temptation to poor compliance, must be of major interest.

Further studies are needed to clarify the effect of various potentially predisposing factors on the response to ketoconazole, and to define more clearly the relapse rate with ketoconazole as compared with effective topical regimens.

Table II. Results of 2 double-blind studies comparing orally administered ketoconazole with miconazole given intravaginally in patients with vaginal candidosis

Treatment (number of patients)[1]	Results[2]									
	at 4 days post-treatment					at 4 weeks post-treatment				
	negative culture	vaginitis	vulvitis	pruritus vulvae	leucor-rhoea	negative culture	vaginitis	vulvitis	pruritus vulvae	leucor-rhoea
Ketoconazole 200mg tid × 3d (108)	91	96	98	77	57	70	88	94	84	55
Miconazole 400mg tid × 3d intravaginally (35)	91	91	94	73	53	81	94	84	66	47
Ketoconazole, as above (30)	96	100		82	62	78	93		75	61
Miconazole, as above (27)	96	92		84	64	96	96		68	60

1 In both studies a matching placebo for oral or intravaginal use was employed to maintain double-blind conditions.
2 Results shown are % of patients with negative cultures or who were symptom-free.

References

Bisschop, M.P.J.M.; Merkus, J.M.W.M.; Scheijgrond, H.; Van Cutsem, J. and van de Kuy, A.: Treatment of vaginal candidiasis with ketoconazole, a new, orally active, antimycotic. European Journal of Obstetrics. Gynecology and Reproductive Biology 9: 253-259 (1979).

Creatsas, G.; Zissis, N.P. and Lolis, D.: Ketoconazole, a new antifungal agent, in vaginal candidiasis. Current Therapeutic Research 28: 121-126 (1980).

del Palacio Hernanz, A.; Coma, A.B.; Sanz Sanz, F.; Guerrero, M.M. and Belaustegui, A.R.-N.: Ketoconazole en candidiasis vulvovaginal. Presented at the 12th Hispano-Lusitanian Congress of Obstetrics and Gynaecology, 1-4 October and 2nd Mediterranean Congress of Chemotherapy, Nice, 13-16 October (1980).

Fregoso-Duenas, F.: Ketoconazole in vulvovaginal candidosis. Reviews of Infectious Diseases 2: 620-624 (1980).

Platts, W.M.: Sexually transmissible diseases; in Avery (Ed) Drug Treatment, 2nd Edition, p.1159-1173 (Adis Press, Sydney and Churchill Livingstone, Edinburgh 1980).

Chapter XII

Chronic Mucocutaneous Candidosis

(figs. 1 and 2)

Chronic mucocutaneous candidosis is likely to occur in individuals with an impaired immune response mechanism (Meinhof, 1979). The disease is difficult to treat, and is often resistant to conventional therapy. When an adequate response does occur it is frequently transient. Multiple foci of infection are often clinically apparent (see fig. 1).

Orally administered ketoconazole has been evaluated in more than 70 patients with chronic mucocutaneous candidosis, including 27 children less than 15 years of age (age range of patients 1 to 62 years) [Arechavala et al., 1980; Drouhet and Dupont, 1980; Graybill et al., 1980; Haneke, 1981; Hay et al., 1980; Kennedy et al., 1981; Kirkpatrick et al., 1980; Morrison and Anderson, 1981; Petersen et al., 1980; Rosenblatt et al., 1980; unpublished data, on file Janssen Research Foundation].

Open Studies

Study Methods

For the major multicentre investigation involving 69 patients, *Candida* was demonstrated in 60 patients at the start of the study; in the remaining 9 the diagnosis was based on historical documentation of candidosis. *Candida albicans* was present in 53 patients and *Candida* sp. in 7 patients. Of those with *C. albicans*, 4 patients were also positive for *Candida parapsilosis*, 2 patients for *Candida guilliermondi* and 1 patient for *Malassezia furfur*. The median duration of the presenting episode of the disease was 6 years (2 weeks to 44 years), and the mean total disease history was 10 years (3 months to 44 years).

58 patients had failed to respond to or did not tolerate previous antifungal therapy, including systemic or topical amphotericin B, miconazole, clotrimazole and nystatin, griseofulvin and other topical antifungal agents. Only intravenous amphotericin B had produced encouraging results, but severe side effects occurred in some patients.

Adult patients usually received a dose of 200mg of ketoconazole once daily with a meal. Children received daily doses of 4.2 to 11.2mg/kg (median 6.7mg/kg).

Table I. Results of ketoconazole treatment in 69 patients with chronic mucocutaneous candidosis

Clinical result	No. of patients (%)	Mycological evidence			Overall results[1]			
		negative	positive	not done	±	+	+ +	+ + +
No change	2 (3)		2					
Moderate improvement	14 (20)	2	5	7				
Marked improvement	34 (49)	7	16	11				
Clinical cure	19 (28)	11	2	6				
All patients	69 (100)	20 (29)	25 (36)	24 (35)	2 (3)	14 (20)	36 (52)	17 (25)

1 ± = no change; + = moderate improvement; + + = marked improvement; + + + = remission.

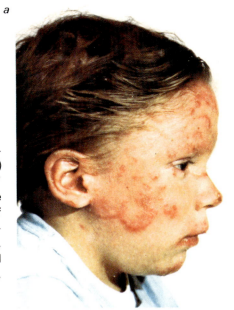
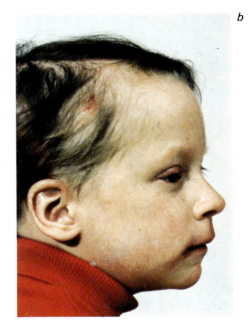

Fig. 1. Chronic mucocutaneous candidosis before (a,c,e)
and after (b,d,f) 5 months'
treatment with ketoconazole
200mg daily. (All plates are of
the same patient) [By courtesy of Dr C.H. Kirkpatrick,
National Jewish Hospital and
Research Center, Denver,
Colorado]

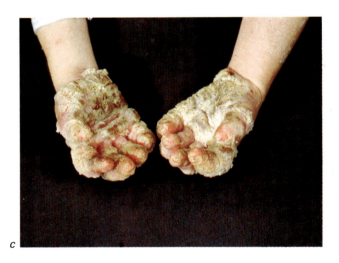
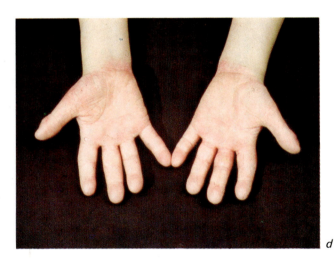

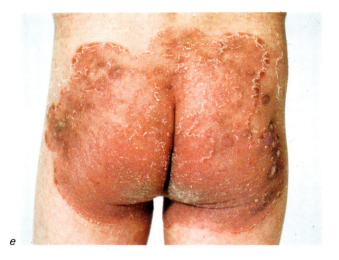
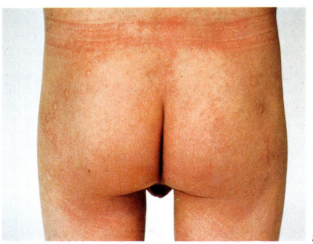

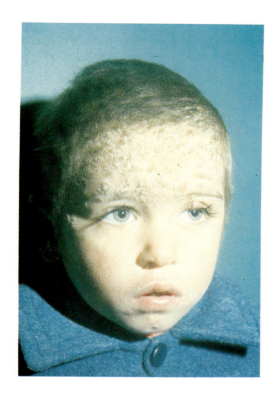

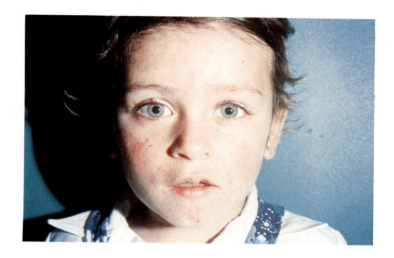

Fig. 2. Results of treatment of 2 patients with chronic mucocutaneous candidosis with ketoconazole 200mg daily for 9 months (top) and 2 months (bottom). [By courtesy of Professor R. Negroni, Catedra de Microbiologia, Parasitologia e Immunologia, Buenos Aires (top) and Dr J. R. Graybill, University of Texas, San Antonio (bottom)]

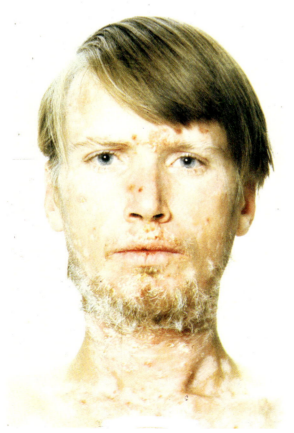

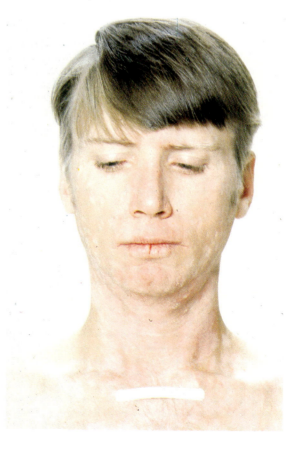

Response to Ketoconazole

Based on clinical and mycological evaluation, with ketoconazole treatment 25% of patients achieved remission, 52% showed marked improvement and 3% were unchanged (table I). The median time to response was about 16 weeks (fig. 3).

Within the time frame of the study (patients evaluated after a median of 18 weeks of treatment), nail lesions were slower to heal than skin or mucosal lesions. Mucosal lesions usually healed within days, skin lesions within weeks to a few months and nail lesions after a variable period of up to several months (Drouhet and Dupont, 1980; Graybill et al., 1980; Peterson et al., 1980). In reporting the results of the multicentre study, patients with nail lesions which were improved, but still present at the time of evaluation, were classed as 'markedly improved' rather than 'cured', suggesting that the overall remission rate may have improved with longer treatment.

Controlled Studies

In a double-blind placebo controlled study in 12 patients with chronic mucocutaneous candidosis ketoconazole was significantly (p = 0.001) superior to placebo treatment (Kirkpatrick et al., 1980; Petersen et al., 1980). Of 6 patients receiving ketoconazole, none had any oral lesions remaining after treatment for 6 months and skin lesions were improved in all patients receiving active drug. Only 1 of 6 placebo-treated patients had any lasting improvement in mouth lesions and none showed beneficial effects on skin involvement. Patients classed as treatment failures (all those receiving placebo) subsequently responded to ketoconazole, and are included in the open study results described above.

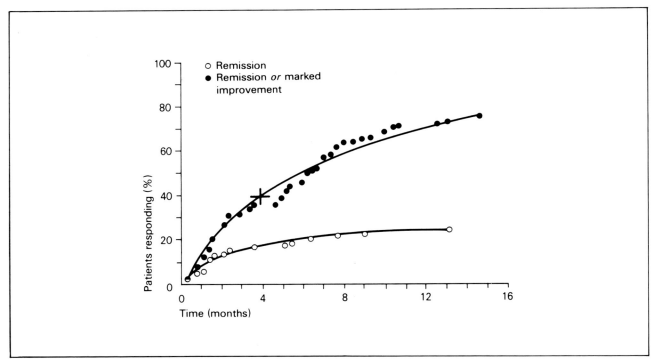

Fig. 3. Time course of response to orally administered ketoconazole of patients with chronic mucocutaneous candidosis. The cross indicates the median time to response.

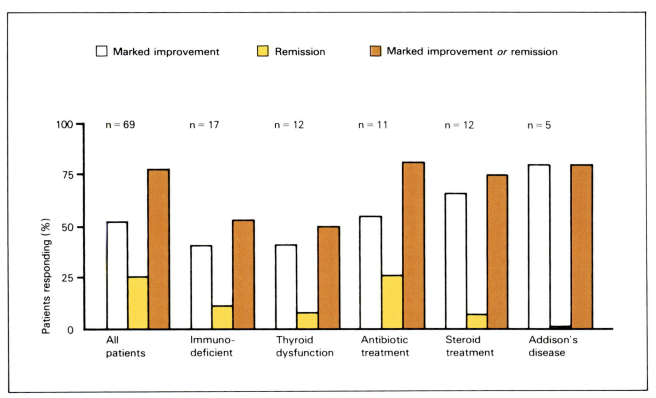

Fig. 4. The effect of possibly predisposing conditions or concomitant disease on the response to ketoconazole of patients with chronic mucocutaneous candidosis.

Factors Affecting Response

Increasing the daily dose above 200mg (to 400mg) did not always improve response rates in adults. Similarly, in chidlren receiving varying daily doses up to 11.2mg/kg/day there was no apparent dose-response relationship. An attempt to reduce the frequency of administration of the daily dose to 3 days weekly was unsuccessful in 3 of 4 patients.

A small number of patients with immunodeficiencies, thyroid dysfunction, or receiving corticosteroids tended to respond less readily than the group as a whole (fig. 4). Interestingly, in a single patient receiving concomitant antacid therapy only moderate improvement occurred, inviting speculation that this may have been due to reduced absorption of ketoconazole (see chapter VI).

Relapse

Three patients in remission were followed for up to 6 months; 1 patient relapsed in the first month of follow-up while the remaining 2 were symptom-free after 2 and 6 months. A small number of patients in remission have continued to receive ketoconazole in intermittent dosage (commonly 200mg every other day) in an effort to prevent relapse (Graybill et al., 1980; Peterson et al., 1980). Relapse did occur in some of these patients, with subsequent improvement on re-instituting daily therapy.

Conclusions

Results with orally administered ketoconazole in patients with chronic mucocutaneous candidosis are encouraging, considering the recalcitrant nature of the disease. Since relapse is a common problem in these patients, in the past often necessitating repeated courses of intravenously administered amphotericin B with the risk of nephrotoxicity, further follow-up data are needed to determine the relapse rate after ketoconazole-induced remission. The benefits of, and optimum dosage for prophylactic therapy also need to be examined further.

References

Arechavala, A.; Finquelievich, J.; Galimberti, R. et al.: Tratamiento con ketoconazol de las candidiasis mucocutaneas cronicas. Revista Argentina de Micologia 3: 16-22 (1980).

Drouhet, E. and Dupont, B.: Chronic mucocutaneous candidosis and other superficial and systemic mycoses successfully treated with ketoconazole. Reviews of Infectious Diseases 2: 606-619 (1980).

Graybill, J.R.; Herndon, J.H.; Kniker, W.T. and Levine, H.B.: Ketoconazole treatment of chronic mucocutaneous candidiasis. Archives of Dermatology 111: 1137-1141 (1980).

Haneke, E.: Ketoconazole treatment of dermatomycoses. International Congress of Chemotherapy, Florence, Italy, 19-24 July (1981).

Hay, R.J.; Wells, R.S.; Clayton, Y.M. and Wingifield, H.J.: Treatment of chronic mucocutaneous candidosis with ketoconazole: a study of 12 cases. Reviews of Infectious Diseases 2: 600-605 (1980).

Kennedy, C.T.C.; Valdimarsson, H. and Hay, R.J.: Chronic mucocutaenous candidiasis with a serum-dependent neutrophil defect: response to ketoconazole. Journal of the Royal Society of Medicine 74: 158-162 (1981).

Kirkpatrick, C.H.; Petersen, E.A. and Alling, D.W.: Treatment of chronic mucocutaneous candidosis with ketoconazole: Preliminary results of a controlled, double-blind clinical trial. Reviews of Infectious Diseases 2: 599 (1980).

Meinhof, W.: Candida-mykosen and cellulare immundefekte. Aentralalatt Fuer Haut und Geschlechtskrank Heiten Sowie Deren Grenzgebiete 141: 1-10 (1979).

Morrison, J.G.L. and Andersen, R.: Familial chronic mucocutaneous candidiasis successfully treated with oral ketoconazole. South African Medical Journal 59: 237-239 (1981).

Petersen, E.A.; Alling, D.W. and Kirkpatrick, C.H.: Treatment of chronic mucocutaneous candidiasis with ketoconazole. A controlled clinical trial. Annals of Internal Medicine 93: 791-795 (1980).

Rosenblatt, H.M.; Byrne, W.; Ament, M.E.; Graybill, J. and Stiehm, E.R.: Successful treatment of mucocutaneous candidiasis with ketoconazole. Journal of Pediatrics 97: 657-660 (1980).

Chapter XIII

Onychomycosis and Perionyxis
(figs. 1-2)

Fungal infection of the nails or the surrounding nail fold presents a difficult therapeutic problem. Although griseofulvin is effective in dermatophytic infections, especially of the fingernails, extended treatment is usually required and this is sometimes accompanied by treatment-limiting side effects such as gastritis, diarrhoea or photosensitivity. Yeast infections are not susceptible to griseofulvin therapy, and traditionally have been treated topically with mixed success.

More than 126 patients with onychomycosis due to dermatophyte or yeast infections, and 7 patients with perionyxis, have been treated with orally administered ketoconazole (Botter et al., 1979; Brugmans et al., 1980; Galimberti et al., 1979, 1980; Haneke, 1981; Robertson et al., 1980; unpublished data, on file Janssen Research Foundation).

Open Studies in Onychomycoses

Study Methods

In a multicentre study 126 patients with mycoses of the fingernails (71 patients) and/or toenails (66 patients) were treated with ketoconazole. At the time of evaluation 115 cases were evaluable. A small number of additional cases have also been studied by individual investigators.

Trichophyton mentagrophytes was cultured in 4 cases, *Trichophyton rubrum* in 63 cases, *Microsporum canis* in 2 cases, *Candida* sp. in 29 cases, *Candida albicans* in 17 cases and *Torulopsis glabrata* and *Aspergillus flavus* once each. The median duration of infection was 3 years for dermatophytes (range of 6 months to 30 years) and 1 year for yeasts (range of 1 month to 11 years); in the patient in whom *Aspergillus* was isolated onychomycosis had been present for 5 years. 43 patients had failed to respond to or had relapsed after previous topical or systemic (griseofulvin) antifungal therapy.

Most patients received a single dose of 200mg of ketoconazole daily, taken with a meal, for 8 to 65 weeks prior to evaluation (median of 22 weeks). A very small number of patients had the dosage increased during the course of treatment to 400 or 800mg daily. Evaluation was based on both clinical and mycological responses.

Results

In the multicentre study 78 of 115 cases achieved remission, marked and moderate improvement occurred in 15 cases each, and no change was seen in 7 cases (table I; fig. 3). Although both fingernail and toenail lesions responded in many cases, toenail lesions took longer to heal; the

Table I. Response rate in 115 cases of onychomycosis treated with orally administered ketoconazole

Clinical results	No. of patients (%)	Mycological evidence			Overall results[1]			
		negative	positive	not done	±	+	+ +	+ + +
No change	7 (6)	5	1	1				
Moderate improvement	15 (13)	7	5	3				
Marked improvement	14 (12)	6	7	1				
Clinical cure	77 (67)	1	43	33				
Not evaluable	2 (2)	0	0	2				
All cases	115 (100)	19 (17)	56 (49)	40 (35)	7 (6)	15 (13)	15 (13)	78 (68)

1 ± = no change; + = moderate improvement; + + = marked improvement, + + + = remission.

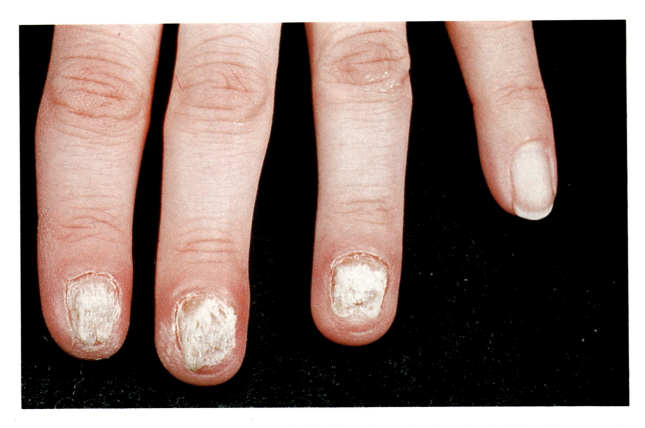

Fig. 1. Response of a patient with onychomycosis (*Candida* sp.) treated with orally administered ketoconazole for 8 months. (By courtesy of Dr R.J. Hay, London School of Hygiene and Tropical Medicine, and the Department of Medical Photography, St. John's Hospital for Diseases of the Skin)

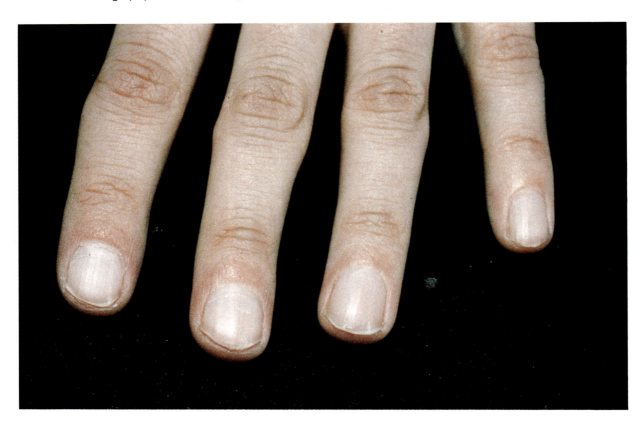

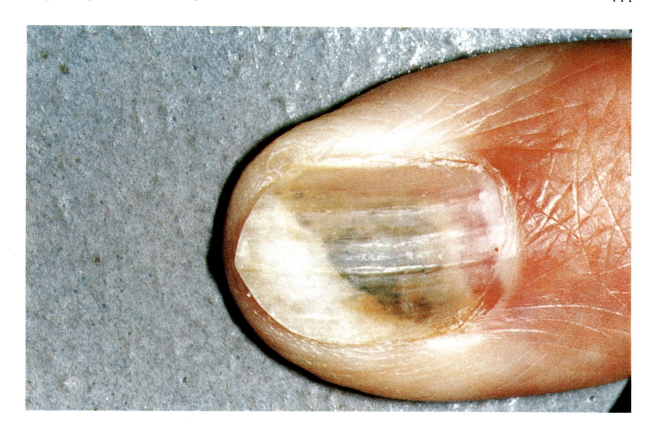

Fig. 2. *Trichophyton rubrum* infection of the nail before and after 7 months' treatment with oral ketoconazole. (By courtesy of Dr A. Englehardt, Hautfacharzt Stationäre Behandlung Hautklinik, Rottweil, Germany)

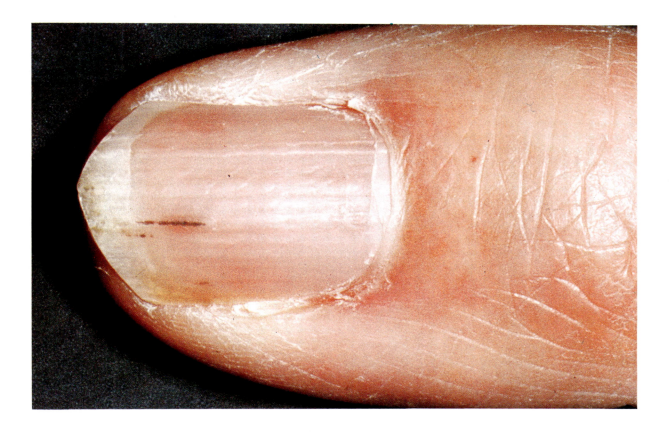

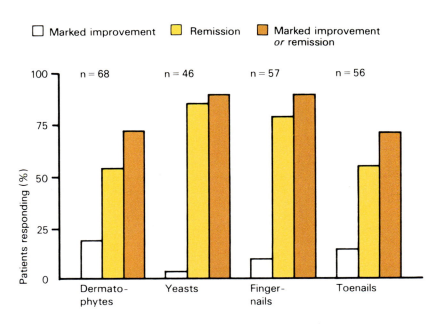

Fig. 3. Response rates in patients with onychomycosis treated with ketoconazole, showing response as a function of the type of infection and site involved.

number of fingernail lesions had decreased by 82% and toenail lesions by 55% at the time of evaluation. Both dermatophyte and yeast infections were improved, but results appeared better for yeast infections (see fig. 3). Yeast infections are more common in fingernails than toenails and fingernails respond to treatment more rapidly; at the time of evaluation many patients had not been treated long enough for toenails to clear. The median time to response was approximately 20 to 25 weeks for all lesions.

In a study conducted entirely in patients with onychomycoses considered to be unresponsive to griseofulvin, all of 16 patients showed definite nail clearing after 6 to 10 weeks of ketoconazole therapy (Robertson et al., 1980). Three of these patients with chronic *T. rubrum* infections (skin and nails) shown in the laboratory to be resistant to griseofulvin responded readily to ketoconazole (see also chapter VIII).

Open Studies in Perionyxis   In 7 patients with perionyxis (*C. albicans* 5 patients, *Candida krusei* and *Candida stellatoidea* 1 patient each) ketoconazole in a single daily dose of 200mg was highly effective. After 3 to 8 weeks of treatment 6 patients were considered to be in remission and 1 patient was markedly improved.

Controlled Studies in Onychomycoses

Preliminary results of a small double-blind comparative study, conducted in patients with dermatophytic onychomycoses using similar diagnostic and evaluation criteria as in the open studies, suggest greater efficacy with ketoconazole 400mg daily than with griseofulvin 500mg daily. However, the small number of patients involved necessitates cautious interpretation of the study results. After 10 to 20 weeks of treatment in 11 evaluable patients, 3 of 6 patients receiving ketoconazole were markedly improved and 3 were moderately improved. Of 5 patients receiving griseofulvin, 1 patient was markedly improved, 2 were moderately improved and 2 remained unchanged. In patients showing the least improvement increasing the dose did not enhance the effect of either drug.

Factors Affecting Response

As discussed above, the site of infection and the infecting fungus were related to the response rates. However, there was no difference in response between patients previously treated with an antifungal drug and those not previously treated, and results were not related to the daily dose of ketoconazole.

Interestingly, in one series 2 of 3 patients who failed to respond had very low ketoconazole plasma concentrations (less than $0.78\mu g/ml$) on several determinations, apparently related to poor absorption as a result of gastrectomy or hypochlorhydria (Galimberti et al., 1980).

Relapse

Most patients treated successfully have not been followed-up to evaluate the longer term effectiveness after discontinuing treatment. No relapse occurred in 3 patients with ketoconazole-induced remissions of toenail infections who were followed for 2 to 6 months (Robertson et al., 1980).

Conclusions

Orally administered ketoconazole is an effective treatment for both dermatophytic and yeast onychomycoses. Its broad spectrum provides a clear advantage over griseofulvin in these conditions, which is effective only in dermatophytic nail infections; preliminary evidence suggests that ketoconazole is at least as effective as griseofulvin in dermatophytic infections, which property, in conjunction with its anticandidal activity, represents an important advance in what has been a most difficult treatment area.

References

Botter, A.A.; Dethier, F.; Mertens, R.L.J.; Morias, J. and Peremans, W.: Skin and nail mycoses: treatment with ketoconazole, a new oral antimycotic agents Mykosen 22: 274-278 (1979).

Brugmans, J.; Scheijgrond, H.; Van Cutsem, J.; Van den Bossche, H.; Baisier, A. and Hörig, Ch.: Orale langzeitbehandlung von onychomykosen mit ketoconazol. Mykosen 23: 405-415 (1980).

Galimberti, R.; Negroni, R.; Iglesia de Elias Costa, M.R. and Casalá, A.M.: Tratamiento de las onicomicosis con ketoconazol. Revista Argentina de Micologia 2: 5-10 (1979).

Galimberti, R.; Negroni, R.; Iglesia de Elias Costa, M.R. and Casala, A.M.: The activity of ketoconazole in the treatment of onychomycosis. Reviews of Infectious Diseases 2: 596-598 (1980).

Haneke, E.: Ketoconazole treatment of dermatomycoses. International Congress of Chemotheapy, Florence, Italy, 19-24 July (1981).

Robertson, M.H.; Hanifin, J.M. and Parker, F.: Oral therapy with ketoconazole for dermatophyte infections unresponsive to griseofulvin. Reviews of Infectious Diseases 2: 578-581 (1980).

Ketoconazole: Clinical Experience in Deep Mycoses

To an even greater degree than in superficial mycoses, where in some instances reasonably effective treatments do exist, the introduction of a new antifungal drug for the treatment of systemic fungal infections is an event of much importance. That the drug can be administered orally in these conditions serves to heighten interest still further. A summary of the efficacy of orally administered ketoconazole in various deep mycoses is shown in table I, with more detailed discussion in chapters XIV to XIX which follow. Clearly, results are highly encouraging in many of these difficult therapeutic areas.

Table I. Summary of the effectiveness of orally administered ketoconazole in some deep mycoses in patients included in the multicentre study

Condition (number of patients)	Response (%)		
	remission	remission or marked improvement	overall efficacy[1]
Systemic candidosis (47)	72	83	+ + +
Candiduria (20)	65		+ +
Paracoccidioidomycosis (75)	79	95	+ + +
Histoplasmosis (31)	52	84	+ + +
Coccidioidomycosis (85)	13	35	+ (+)
Chromomycosis (17)	24	53	+ +

1   + + + = highly effective; + + = moderately effective; + = effectiveness doubtful

Chapter XIV

Systemic Candidosis and Candiduria

Systemic candidosis is a fungal disease encountered particularly in debilitated patients or those in whom predisposing circumstances are present, such as immunodeficiency, diabetes, aggressive corticosteroid, cytostatic or broad spectrum antibiotic therapy, or indwelling venous or urinary catheters (p.7). In addition deep focal invasion of *Candida* sp. may occur in a number of sites including bladder, peritoneum and oesophagus. Such cases normally carry a better prognosis but, in most instances, require chemotherapy.

47 patients with deep or systemic candidosis: infections of the bladder (27 patients), upper urinary tract (6 patients), respiratory tract (7 patients), oesophagus (3 patients), musculoskeletal system (1 patient) and those with disseminated foci (3 patients), as well as 20 patients with asymptomatic candiduria, have been treated with orally administered ketoconazole (Borelli et al., 1979; Weisburd and Bonazzola, 1979; unpublished data, on file Janssen Research Foundation).

Open Studies in Systemic Candidosis

Study Methods

Diagnosis was by culture of *Candida* from all patients, as well as by biopsy, serology studies, x-rays or endoscopy in some cases. *Candida* sp. was cultured from 33 patients, *Candida albicans* from 9 patients and *Candida tropicalis* from 5 patients. The median duration of the candidal infection was 2 years and of the presenting episode 1 year (range of 1 week to 10 years in both cases). 9 patients had previously been treated with antifungal agents, usually with several over a period of time, including intravenously administered amphotericin B, miconazole given intravenously, orally or used topically, nystatin given orally, flucytosine or natamycin; 7 patients failed to respond to or relapsed after previous treatment.

Results

Patients were given ketoconazole 200mg once or twice daily with a meal for a median of 10 days (range of 3 to 201 days) before evaluation, which was based on clinical and mycological response.

Remission occurred in 72% of patients, marked improvement in 11% and no change was seen in 17% (table I). The median time to response was about 1 week (fig. 1). In addition to those conditions described in the table, ketoconazole has been administered to a patient with fungal endocarditis due to *Candida parapsilosis* (Samelson et al., 1980). The patient had relapsed after 7 years of suppressive therapy with flucytosine. She received intravenous amphotericin B (total dose of 2.4g) and then ketoconazole 400mg/day given orally, and remained well during 12 weeks on this regimen.

Table I. Results of treatment of 47 patients with systemic candidosis with orally administered ketoconazole

Clinical results	No. of patients (%)	Mycological evidence			Overall results[1]			
		negative	positive	not done	±	+	+ +	+ + +
No change	8 (17)	4	4					
Moderate improvement	0							
Marked improvement	5 (11)	1		4				
Clinical cure	33 (70)	32		1				
Not evaluable	1 (2)	1						
All patients	47 (100)	38 (81)	4 (8)	5 (11)	8 (17)		5 (11)	34 (72)

1 ± = no change; + = moderate improvement; + + = marked improvement; + + + = remission.

2 of 34 patients in remission received ketoconazole prophylactically to prevent relapse. Of the 32 patients who discontinued treatment, 10 who were followed up for 1 month remained in remission.

Open Studies in Candiduria

Study Methods

20 patients with asymptomatic candiduria related to chronic debilitating disease, immunological defects, aggressive corticosteroid or antibiotic therapy, catheters or prostheses have been treated with orally administered ketoconazole. *Candida* was demonstrated in urine cultures of all patients; *Candida* sp. in 12 patients, *C. albicans* in 5 patients, *Candida krusei* in 2 patients and *C. tropicalis* in 1 patient.

Treatment was with a dose of 200mg once or twice daily with a meal. Urine cultures were repeated after a median of 14 days of treatment (range of 11 to 78 days).

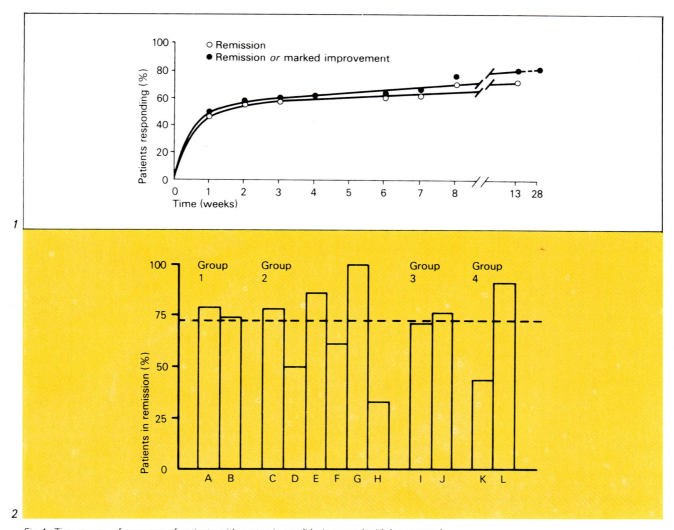

Fig. 1. Time course of response of patients with systemic candidosis treated with ketoconazole.

Fig. 2. Remission rates in various groups of patients with systemic candidosis compared with the group as a whole (dashed line). Group 1 (n = 47) — duration of infection: A = < 6 months, B = > 6 months; Group 2 — location of infection: C = bladder (n = 27), D = upper urinary tract (n = 6), E = respiratory tract (n = 7), F = oesophagus (n = 3), G = musculoskeletal (n = 1), H = generalised (n = 3); Group 3 (n = 47) — ketoconazole dosage: I = < 200mg daily, J = > 200mg daily; Group 4 (n = 47) previous antifungal treatment: K = yes, L = no. See also text.

Results

13 patients (65%) had negative urine cultures at the end of treatment. The median time to negative urine culture was about 1 week in responding patients.

Factors Affecting Response

In patients with candiduria the response rate in males (86%) tended to be higher than in females (54%), but the difference was not statistically significant in this small group. In patients with deep or systemic candidosis some subgroups responded better than others (fig. 2), but again the differences were not statistically significant; obviously such data must be interpreted cautiously considering the small numbers of patients involved. It is of interest that 6 of 8 patients with systemic candidosis who did not respond to ketoconazole were diabetic patients.

Conclusions

Orally administered ketoconazole is an effective treatment for certain forms of deep or systemic candidosis including candiduria. However, the real value of ketoconazole in such infections and, in particular, whether some patients are more likely to respond than others cannot be clearly defined until data has become available from a larger number of patients. In addition it would be important to know the extent of *Candida* colonisation in individual patients as this may have considerable bearing upon the results of treatment.

References

Borelli, D.; Fuentes, J.; Leiderman, E.; Restrepo-M.A.; Bran, J.L.; Legendre, R.; Levine, H.B. and Stevens, D.A.: Ketoconazole, an oral antifungal: laboratory and clinical assessment of imidazole drugs. Postgraduate Medical Journal 55: 657-661 (1979).

Samelson, L.E.; Lerner, S.A.; Resnekov, L. and Anagnostopoulos, C.: Relapse of *Candida parapsilosis* endocarditis after long-term suppression with flucytosine: retreatment with valve replacement and ketoconazole. Annals of Internal Medicine 93: 838-839 (1980).

Weisburd, G.J. and Bonazzola, R.: R 41 400, ketoconazole, en el tratamiento de las micosis profundas. IX Jornadas Argentinas de Micologia, Resistencia, Chaco, Rep. Argentina, July 31-August 4 (1979).

Chapter XV

Paracoccidioido-mycosis (South American Blastomycosis)
(figs. 1-3)

Paracoccidioidomycosis, a fungal infection due to *Paracoccidioides brasiliensis* which may present as involving primarily the skin and mucous membranes or the lungs or other viscera, is endemic in some regions of South and Central America. If untreated the disease generally follows a progressive, fatal course. Sulphonamides offer suppressive but probably not curative treatment. Intravenously administered amphotericin B is effective, but relapse occurs frequently. Miconazole is effective since *P. brasilienis* is very sensitive to it; indeed paracoccidioidomycosis is the only systemic mycosis that can be treated with oral miconazole.

More than 75 patients with paracoccidioidomycosis have been treated with orally administered ketoconazole (Borelli et al., 1979; Cucé et al., 1980; Del Negro (1979); Negroni et al., 1979, 1980; Restrepo et al., 1980 and in press; Weisburd and Bonazzola, 1979; unpublished data, on file Janssen Research Foundation).

Open Studies

Study Methods

In the major multicentre study of ketoconazole in paracoccidioidomycosis 75 patients were treated by 6 investigators. Diagnosis was by culture of *P. brasiliensis* in all patients except one whose infection was historically documented, and by serology, x-ray, endoscopy or animal inoculation methods in some cases. 40 patients had more than one organ or system affected.

The median duration of the disease was 12 months (range of 14 weeks to 23 years) and of the presenting episode 6 months (range of 1 week to 16 years). 39 patients had previously failed to respond to, or relapsed after, treatment with amphotericin B given intravenously, miconazole given intravenously or orally, clotrimazole given orally or sulphonamides.

Most patients were treated with ketoconazole 200mg given once or twice daily with meals, for a median treatment period of 10 weeks (range of 3 to 55 weeks). Evaluation was based on clinical and mycological responses, or in some patients on clinical results and serological testing.

Results

79% of patients were judged to be in remission, 16% were markedly improved, 4% were moderately improved and a single patient was unchanged after treatment with ketoconazole (table I). The median time to

Table I. Response in 75 patients with paracoccidioidomycosis treated with orally administered ketoconazole

Clinical results	No. of patients (%)	Mycological results			Serological results[1]				Overall results[2]			
		nega-tive	no change	not done	nega-tive	resi-dual	no change	not done	±	+	+ +	+ + +
No change	1 (1)						1 (1)					
Moderate improvement	3 (4)					1 (1)	2 (3)					
Marked improvement	11 (15)					6 (8)	3 (4)	2 (3)				
Clinical cure	60 (80)				9 (12)	34 (45)	1 (1)	16 (21)				
All patients	75 (100)	18 (24)	7 (9)	50 (67)	9 (12)	41 (55)	7 (9)	18 (24)	1 (1)	3 (4)	12 (16)	59 (79)

1 Based on specific antibodies in serum, or in a few patients CSF. 'Residual' indicates antibody titre decreased by at least 2 dilutions, but still positive.
2 ± = no change; + = moderate improvement; + + = marked improvement; + + + = remission.

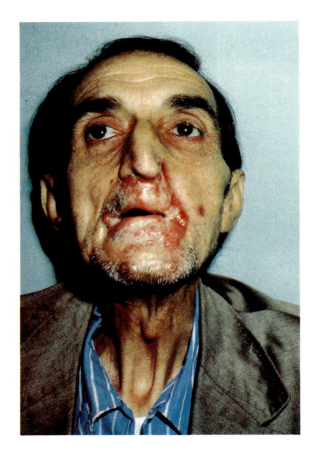

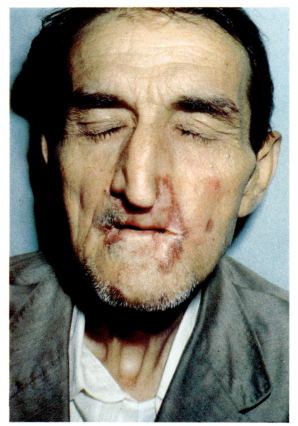

Fig. 1. A patient with para-coccidioidomycosis before and after treatment with ketoconazole for 2 months (By courtesy of Dr L.C. Cucé, University of Sao Paulo, Brazil).

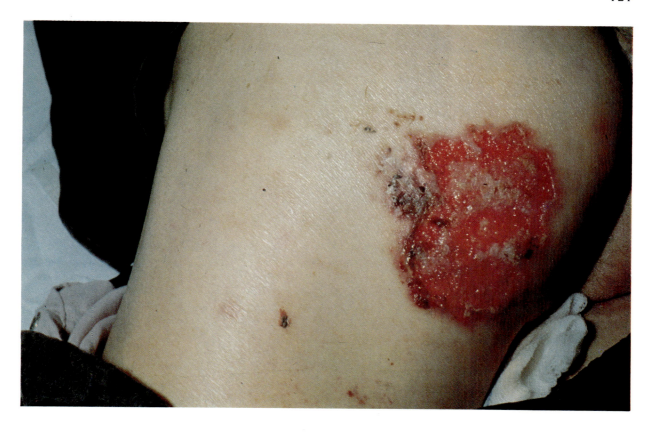

Fig. 2. Paracoccidioidomycosis before and after treatment with ketoconazole for 3 months (By courtesy of Dr L.C. Cucé, University of Sao Paulo, Brazil).

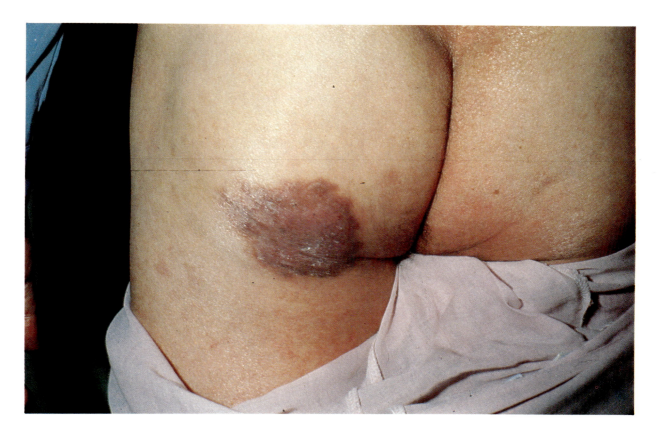

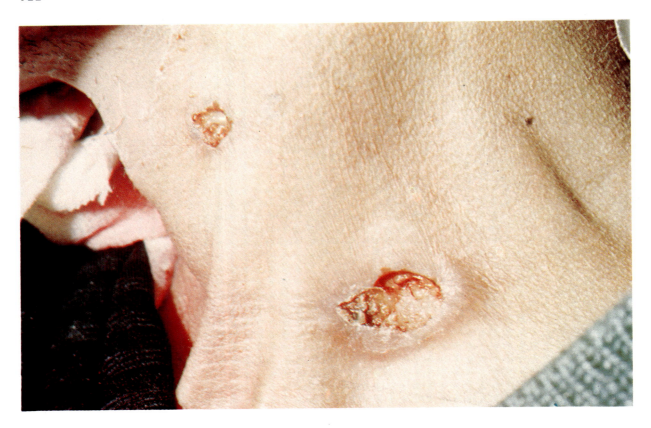

Fig. 3. Paracoccidioidomycosis in a patient before and after treatment with ketoconazole for 3 months (By courtesy of Professor R. Negroni, Catedra de Microbiologia, Parasitologia e Immunologia, Buenos Aires).

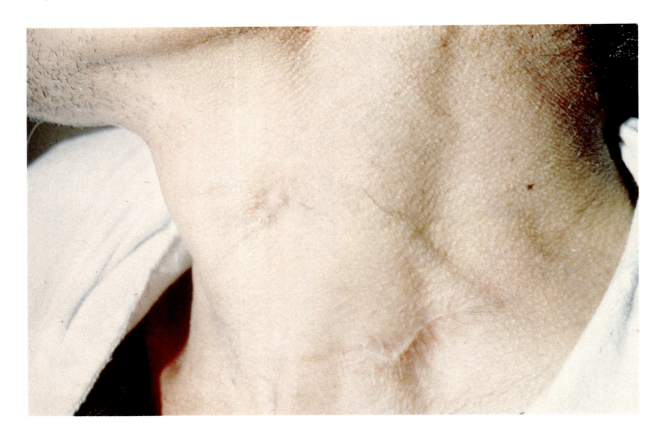

response was 10 weeks (fig. 4). Skin and mucosal lesions healed most rapidly, with obvious improvement within 2 weeks of starting therapy in many patients (Restrepo et al., 1980). Indeed, marked improvement occurred in all organ lesions, although on the basis of x-ray examination pulmonary lesions were less likely to clear completely than those in other organ systems. Thus, the number of lesions in the eye, gastrointestinal tract, haematopoietic or lymphatic systems, upper respiratory tract, head and neck or on the skin was reduced by 88 to 100%, while pulmonary lesions were decreased by 68%. Pulmonary lesions which did heal often left residual fibrotic areas (Restrepo et al., 1980). Whether remaining pulmonary lesions in such patients, as seen on x-ray after treatment, are still active is difficult to determine.

Factors Affecting Response

Neither the type and duration of infection, the dose of ketoconazole, prior antifungal therapy nor, in a small number of patients, concurrent diseases such as Addison's disease, thyroid dysfunction or renal failure or other concurrent drug treatment such as corticosteroid or antibiotic therapy influenced the response to ketoconazole (fig. 5).

Relapse

Of 40 patients who discontinued treatment after achieving remission, 14 were followed up; 11 remained in remission during a follow-up period of 1 to 8 months (median of 2 months). 2 patients relapsed in the first month after therapy terminated and 1 patient in the third month.

A small number of patients have received long term prophylactic therapy with ketoconazole to prevent relapse. In one small series (5 patients), halving the dose after 6 months of treatment to 100mg daily did not result in any relapses (Restrepo et al., 1980). In a second series in which 14

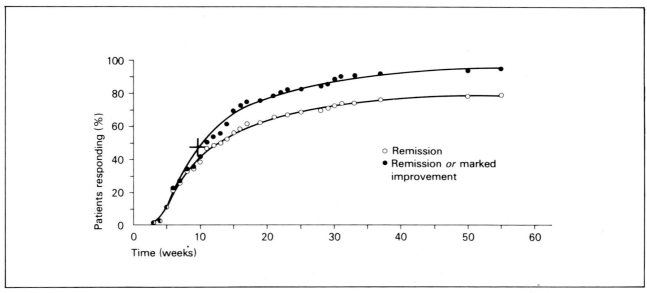

Fig. 4. Response of paracoccidioidomycosis to ketoconazole. Time course of response in 75 patients. The cross indicates the median.

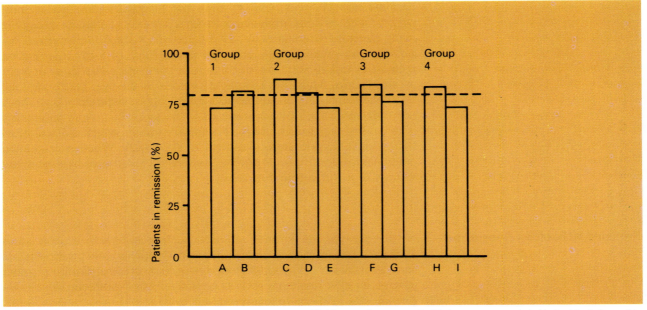

Fig. 5. Remission rates in various sub-groups of patients with paracoccidioidomycosis compared with the group as a whole (dashed line). Group 1 (n = 75) — recent versus old infections: A = ≤ 6 months, B = > 6 months. Group 2 — type of infection: C = localised (n = 35), D = 1 affected organ or system but with multiple sites, E = disseminated. Group 3 (n = 75) — ketoconazole dose: F = ≤ 200mg daily, G = > 200mg daily. Group 4 (n = 75) = previous antifungal treatment: H = yes, I = no.

patients were treated for 90 days only (400mg daily for 30 days, then 200mg daily for 60 days), and 23 other patients were continued on treatment after 90 days with a further dosage reduction to 200mg 3 times weekly, continued administration reduced the occurrence of relapses, but 2 patients receiving continued therapy did relapse during a 10-month follow-up period (relapse rates of 50% and 9% without and with continued treatment, respectively) [Cucé et al., unpublished].

Conclusion

Ketoconazole clearly has considerable potential in the treatment of paracoccidioidomycosis. If wider clinical experience confirms the experiences described above it seems likely that ketoconazole may become the 'agent of choice' in this disease. The optimum duration of initial treatment, and the optimum dosage and duration for prophylactic treatment following the achievement of remission, remain to be clarified. Comparative studies with amphotericin B and possibly sulphonamides, using either historical or, preferably, concurrent controls, would be of great interest.

Before the 'true' relapse rate of paracoccidioidomycosis after ketoconazole therapy can be clearly stated an adequate number of patients must be followed up for an extended period, probably for 5 years or more. The difficulties in gathering such data are obvious.

References

Borelli, D.; Fuentes, J.; Leiderman, E.; Restrepo-M.A.; Bran, J.L.; Legendre, R.; Levine, H.B. and Stevens, D.A.: Ketoconazole, an oral antifungal: laboratory and clinical assessment of imidazole drug. Postgraduate Medical Journal 55: 657-661 (1979).
Cucé, L.C.; Wroclawski, E.L. and Sampaio, S.A.P.: Treatment of paracoccidioidomycosis, candidiasis, chromomycosis, lobomycosis and mycetoma with ketoconazole. International Journal of Dermatology 19: 405-408 (1980).

Del Negro, G.: Clinical and seriologic trial with a new imidazole derivative in extra-cutaneous forms of paracoccidioidomycosis. Preliminary results. First International Symposium on Ketoconazole, Medellin, Colombia (1979).

Negroni, R.; Gonzalez Montaner, L.J.; Palma Beltran, O.; Tuculet, M.A. and Rey, D.: Resultados del ketoconazol (R 41400) en el tratamiento de la paracoccidioido-micosis y la histoplasmosis. Revista Argentina de Micologia 2: 12-18 (1979).

Negroni, R.; Robles, A.M.; Arechavala, A.; Tuculet, M.A. and Galimberti, R.: Ketoconazole in the treatment of paracoccidioidomycosis and histoplasmosis. Reviews of Infectious Diseases 2: 643-649 (1980).

Restrepo, A.; Stevens, D.A.; Gomez, I.; Leiderman, E.; Angel, R.; Fuentes, J.; Arana, A.; Mejiá, G.; Vanegas, A.C. and Robledo, M.: Ketoconazole: a new drug for the treatment of paracoccidioidomycosis. Reviews of Infectious Diseases 2: 633-642 (1980).

Restrepo, A.; Stevens, D.A.; Leiderman, E.; Fuentes, J.; Arana, A.; Angel, R.; Mejiá, G. and Gomez, I.: Ketoconazole on paracoccidioidomycosis: efficacy of proionged oral therapy. Mycopathologia 72: 35-45 (1980).

Weisburd, G.J. and Bonazzola, R.: R 41400, ketoconazol, en el tratamiento de las micosis profundas, IX jornadas Argentinas de Micologia, Resistancia, Chaco, Argentina, July 31-August 4 (1979).

Chapter XVI

Histoplasmosis
(figs. 1 and 2)

Histoplasmosis, caused by the dimorphic fungus *Histoplasma capsulatum*, is a systemic mycosis which may present as an acute or chronic pulmonary disease or, less commonly, may follow an acute or chronic disseminated course (p.10). Intravenously administered amphotericin B is often effective subject to potential toxicity and the difficulties inherent in intravenous administration of the drug.

More than 30 patients with histoplasmosis have been treated with orally administered ketoconazole (Borelli et al., 1979; Drouhet and Dupont, 1980; Graybill et al., 1979; Lundberg et al., 1979; Negroni et al., 1979, 1980; Reinarz et al., 1980; Weisburd and Bonazzola, 1979; Zellweger, 1981; unpublished data, on file Janssen Research Foundation).

Open Studies

Study Methods

In a multicentre study involving 10 investigators treatment with orally administered ketoconazole was evaluated in 31 patients with histoplasmosis, most with pulmonary or gastrointestinal lesions. *H. capsulatum* was demonstrated in all patients. 16 patients had only one organ or system affected and 12 patients had disseminated disease.

The median duration of the disease was 9 months (range of 1 month to 11 years) and of the presenting episode 5.5 months (range of 1 month to 3 years). 14 patients had failed to respond to or had relapsed after previous antifungal treatment, or had been intolerant of previous treatment; prior agents used were intravenous amphotericin B or miconazole, or orally administered clotrimazole, sulphamethoxazole/trimethoprim or other sulphonamides.

Patients usually received ketoconazole 200mg once or twice daily taken with a meal. Evaluation, based on clinical, serological and mycological responses, took place after a median treatment period of 12 weeks.

Results

Remission was achieved in 52% of patients and marked improvement in 32% (table I). Moderate improvement occurred in 2 patients and no change was seen in 3 patients (10%). (These 5 patients showing no change

Table I. Response in 31 patients with histoplasmosis treated with orally administered ketoconazole

Clinical results	No. patients (%)	Mycological results			Serological results[1]				Overall results[2]			
		negative	no change	not done	negative	residual	no change	not done	±	+	+ +	+ + +
No change	3 (10)					1 (3)	1 (3)	1 (3)				
Moderate improvement	2 (6)				1 (3)			1 (3)				
Marked improvement	10 (32)					4 (13)		6 (19)				
Clinical cure	16 (52)				4 (13)	5 (16)		7 (23)				
All patients	31 (100)	7 (23)	1 (3)	23 (74)	5 (16)	10 (32)	1 (3)	15 (48)	3 (10)	2 (6)	10 (32)	16 (52)

1 Based on specific antibodies in serum, or in 1 patient in CSF. 'Residual' indicates antibody titre decreased by at least 2 dilutions, but still positive.
2 ± = no change; + = moderate improvement; + + = marked improvement; + + + = remission.

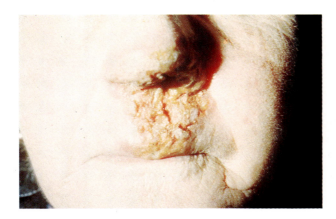

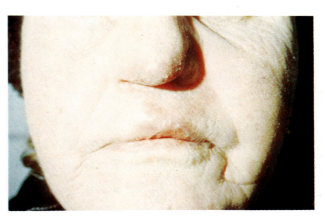

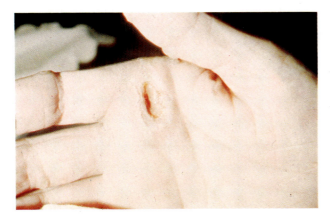

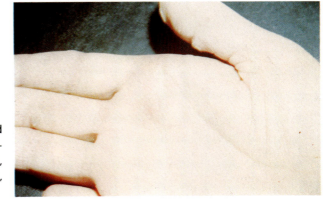

Fig. 1. Histoplasmosis lesions in a patient before (left) and after (right) treatment with orally administered ketoconazole for 3 months. (By courtesy of Professor R. Negroni, Catedra de Microbiologia, Parasitologia e Immunologia, Buenos Aires).

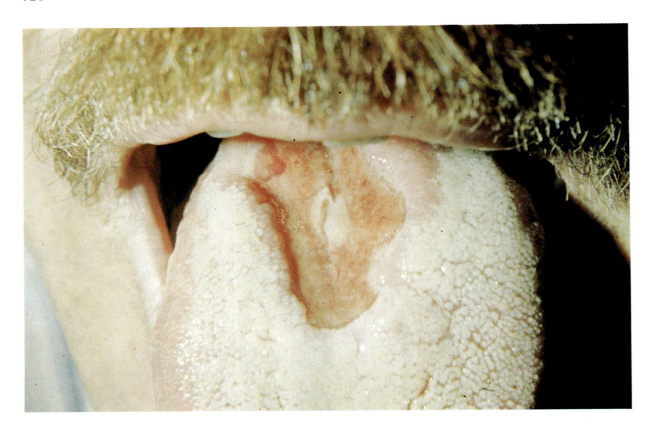

Fig. 2. Histoplasmosis before and after 2 months of treatment with orally administered ketoconazole. (By courtesy of Professor R. Negroni, Catedra de Microbiologia, Parasitologia e Immunologia, Buenos Aires).

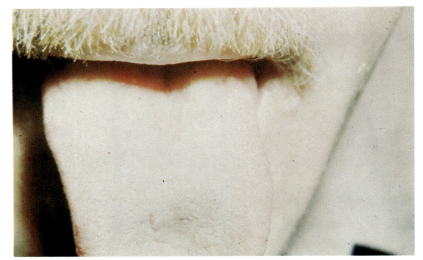

Table II. Effect of ketoconazole treatment on lesions at some sites in patients with histo-plasmosis (see also text)

Site of lesion	Number of pre-treatment lesions	Reduction in number of lesions (%)
Lungs	18	39
Gastrointestinal tract	16	87
Upper respiratory	7	100
Haematopoietic or lymphatic systems	6	60
Musculoskeletal	3	50
Skin	2	100

or only moderate improvement had localised pulmonary lesions which were of long-standing in 4 cases). The median time to remission or marked improvement was about 10 weeks (fig. 3).

Lesions in the gastrointestinal tract or upper respiratory tract responded particularly well (table II). In patients with pulmonary involvement residual lesions were often present on x-ray after treatment, but whether such lesions were active is unclear. In addition to those listed in the table, single lesions in the kidney, eye or head and neck and a single case of meningitis failed to resolve, while 2 patients with a 'febrile reaction' and 1 case of septicaemia did respond.

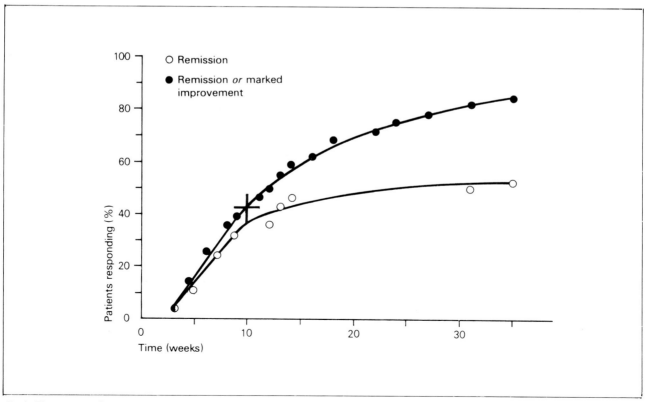

Fig. 3. Time course of response of patients with histoplasmosis to orally administered ketoconazole. The cross indicates the median.

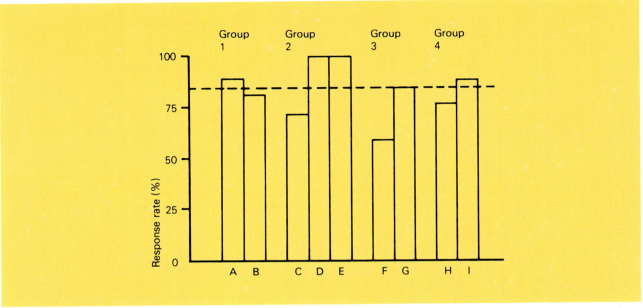

Fig. 4. Response (remission or marked improvement) of various groups of patients with histoplasmosis, compared with the group as a whole [n = 31] (dashed line). Group 1 Duration of infection: A = ≤ 6 months, B = > 6 months; Group 2 — Type of infection: C = 1 site only, D = 1 organ or system with multiple infection sites, E = more than 1 organ or system; Group 3 — Ketoconazole dose: F = ≤ 200mg daily, G = 200mg daily; Group 4 = Previous antifungal therapy: H = yes, I = no.

Factors Influencing Response

As discussed above, lesions at some sites tended to resolve more readily than those at others. Other factors did not appear to influence the response rate, although patients receiving 'higher' doses of ketoconazole showed a tendency toward a greater overall response than those treated with 'lower' doses (fig. 4).

Relapse

6 of 16 patients in remission continued ketoconazole treatment prophylactically. 2 patients who discontinued treatment were followed-up for 3 to 6 months and they remained in remission.

Conclusions

Ketoconazole appears to represent effective oral therapy for histoplasmosis. As in some other areas of use additional follow-up data are needed to evaluate the likelihood of relapse after ketoconazole-induced remission, especially with respect to the significance of residual post-treatment pulmonary lesions seen in many patients with pulmonary involvement.

References

Borelli, D.; Bran, J.L.; Fuentes, J.; Legendre, R.; Leiderman, E.; Levine, H.B.; Restrepo-M.A. and Stevens, D.A.: Ketoconazole, an oral antifungal: laboratory and clinical assessment of imidazole drugs. Postgraduate Medical Journal 55: 657-661 (1979).
Drouhet, E. and Dupont, B.: Chronic mucocutaneous candidosis and other superficial and systemic mycoses successfully treated by ketoconazole. Reviews of Infectious Diseases 2: 606-619 (1980).

Graybill, J.R.; Levine, H.B.; Herndon, J.H. and Kniker, W.T.: Treatment of chronic mucocutaneous candidiasis (CMC) with ketoconazole (KTZ). 11th International Congress of Chemotherapy and 19th Interscience Conference on Antimicrobial Agents and Chemotherapy, Boston, Mass. 1-5 October (1979).

Lundberg, D.; Graybill, R.; Donovan, W.; Levine, H.B.; Drutz, D.J. and Diaz, M.: Clinical evaluation of ketoconazole (KTZ) in the treatment of systemic fungal infections. 11th International Congress of Chemotherapy and 19th Interscience Conference on Antimicrobial Agents and Chemotherapy, Boston, Mass. 1-5 October (1979).

Negroni, R.; Gonzalez Montaner, L.J.; Palma Beltran, O.; Tuculet, M.A. and Rey, D.: Resultados del ketoconazol (R 41400) en el tratamiento de la paracoccidioidomicosis y la histoplasmosis. Revista Argentina de Micologia 2: 12-18 (1979).

Negroni, R.; Robles, A.M.; Arechavala, A.; Tuculet, M.A. and Galimberti, R.: Ketoconazole in the treatment of paracoccidioidomycosis and histoplasmosis. Reviews of Infectious Diseases 2: 643-649 (1980).

Reinarz, J.A.; Mader, J.T. and Masek, J.L.: Ketoconazole therapy for disseminated histoplasmosis. Presented at 20th Interscience Conference on Antimicrobial Agents and Chemotherapy, New Orleans, Louisiana, 22-24 September (1980).

Weisburd, G.J. and Bonazzola, R.: R 41 400, ketoconazol, en el tratamiento de las micosis profundas. IX Jornadas Argentinas de Micologia, Resistencia, Chaco, Argentina 31 July-4 August (1979).

Zellweger, J.P.: Traitement oral au ketoconazole d'un cas d'histoplasmose pulmonaire. Schweizerische Medizinische Wochenschrift 111: 190-191 (1980).

Chapter XVII

Coccidioido-
mycosis

Coccidioidomycosis is an infectious fungal disease caused by the dimorphic fungus *Coccidioides immitis*. It may present as primary coccidioidomycosis, which is normally a self-limiting respiratory infection, or progressive coccidioidomycosis, a chronic disseminated disease which may involve many organ systems including cutaneous and subcutaneous tissue, the viscera or bones (Conant et al., 1971) [p.10]. Although intravenously administered amphotericin B is effective in some patients, failures occur frequently, and nephrotoxicity may prevent an adequate duration of treatment. Similarly, miconazole given intravenously has been of variable effectiveness in small groups of patients (Heel et al., 1980).

Orally administered ketoconazole has been studied in more than 100 patients with coccidioidomycosis (Borelli et al., 1979; Brass et al., 1980; Graybill et al., 1980; Stiller et al., 1980; Welsh et al., 1980; unpublished data, on file Janssen Research Foundation).

Open Studies

Study Methods

In the major multicentre study 94 evaluable patients with coccidioidomycosis were treated with ketoconazole by 11 investigators using a common protocol. (Additional patients have subsequently been treated, bringing the total to more than 100). *C. immitis* was demonstrated in 70 patients, and the infection was historically documented in 14. Other diagnostic methods included serology, x-rays, scans, endoscopy and CSF examination in some patients.

The median duration of the disease was 23 months (range of 2 weeks to 34 years) and of the presenting episode 6 months (range of 1 week to 18 years). 20 patients had more than 1 organ or system affected.

46 patients had failed to respond to or had relapsed after previous antifungal treatment, usually with intravenous amphotericin B or miconazole.

Treatment was usually with ketoconazole 200mg given once or twice daily, for a median treatment period of 26 weeks (range of 8 to 62 weeks). Evaluation was based on both clinical and mycological response.

Table I. Results in 84 patients (85 cases) with coccidioidomycosis of treatment with orally administered ketoconazole

Clinical results	No. of patients (%)	Mycological results			Serological results[1]				Overall results[2]			
		nega-tive	no change	not done	nega-tive	resi-dual	no change	not done	±	+	+ +	+ + +
No change	14 (17)					2 (2)	8 (9)	4 (5)				
Moderate improvement	41 (48)				3 (4)	22 (26)	10 (11)	6 (7)				
Marked improvement	19 (22)				1 (1)	12 (14)	4 (5)	2 (2)				
Clinical cure	11 (13)				2 (2)	5 (6)		4 (5)				
All patients	85 (100)	24 (28)	22 (26)	39 (46)	6 (7)	41 (48)	22 (26)	16 (19)	14 (17)	41 (48)	19 (22)	11 (13)

1 Based on specific antibodies in serum, or in a few patients in CSF. 'Residual' indicates antibody titre decreased by at least 2 dilutions, but still positive.

2 ± = no change; + = moderate improvement; + + = marked improvement; + + + = remission.

Results

Remission occurred in 13% of cases, marked improvement in 22%, moderate improvement in 48% and no change was seen in 17% (table I). The median time to response was about 23 weeks (fig. 1). When results with ketoconazole given orally (200 to 400mg once daily) were compared with those in an approximately comparable group of patients previously treated by the same authors with intravenous miconazole (usually 1000mg 3 times a day), ketoconazole was at least as effective as the intravenous therapy (Stiller et al., 1980); indeed in some analyses ketoconazole was superior to miconazole.

The number of lesions in various organ systems was often too small to make a meaningful statement on the relative response rate related to the focus of infection; however 40% of 47 skin lesions healed during treatment, as did 21% of 14 musculoskeletal lesions, 20% of 5 lesions involving the haematopoietic or lymphatic systems, and 25% of 4 lesions of the head and neck. Most of 47 pulmonary lesions were still detectable on x-ray after treatment, but whether such lesions were then active is not known. No change was seen in a small number of lesions of the eye, the upper respiratory tract or the central nervous system. (In the latter situation, meningitis persisted in 1 patient despite concomitant treatment with orally administered ketoconazole and intrathecally administered amphotericin B). Although 2 kidney lesions were not improved during treatment, 3 renal transplant patients with coccidioiduria (and other involved sites) had clear urine after treatment (De Felice et al., 1980).

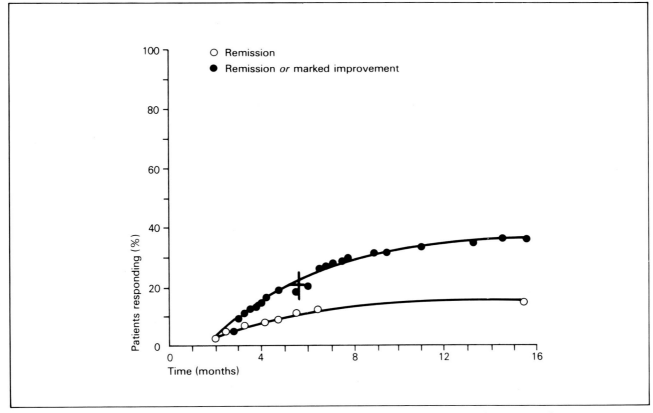

Fig. 1. Coccidioidomycosis treated with ketoconazole. Time course of response to treatment. The cross indicates the median.

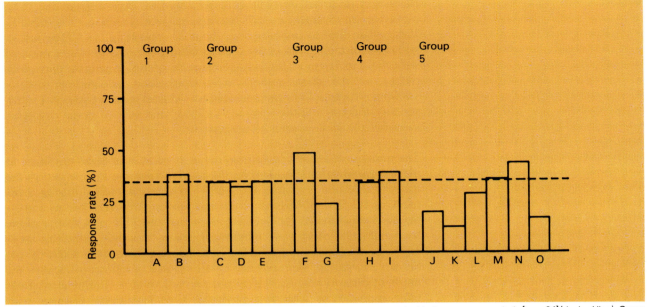

Fig. 2. Remission rates in various sub-groups of patients with coccidioidomycosis compared with the group as a whole [n = 84] (dashed line). Group 1 — Duration of infection: A = ⩽ 6 months, B = > 6 months; Group 2 — Type of infection: C = 1 infection site only; D = 1 organ or system with multiple infection sites; E = more than 1 organ system; Group 3 — Ketoconazole dose: F = ⩽ 200mg daily, G = > 200mg daily; Group 4 — Previous antifungal therapy: H = yes, I = no; Group 5 — Other particular conditions: J = immunodeficiency, K = diabetes mellitus, L = corticosteroid therapy, M = antibiotic therapy, N = renal failure, O = cimetidine and antacid therapy.

Factors Affecting Response

The outcome of treatment did not appear to be affected by the duration of infection, the dosage of ketoconazole used, previous antifungal therapy or most other 'particular conditions' (fig. 2), although a small number of patients with diabetes mellitus or immunodeficiencies tended to respond poorly. As mentioned above, coccidioidal meningitis may be less amenable to therapy than other forms of the disease.

Relapse

Little follow-up data is available to document the incidence of relapse. Of 8 patients in remission followed-up for varying periods, 1 patient had a relapse in the first month after treatment but subsequently achieved a second remission with ketoconazole therapy.

Conclusions

Coccidioidomycosis is a condition which is difficult to treat and this is reflected in the *relatively* low remission rate with ketoconazole therapy compared with that following ketoconazole treatment of other fungal diseases. Nevertheless, the results reported here are encouraging and indicate that ketoconazole may have an important role in the therapy of this infection; but clearly more data are needed before the place of the drug in therapy can be accurately stated. Additional follow-up data to determine the likelihood of relapse, and the merits of 'longer term' treatment, must be awaited. A well designed comparative study with amphotericin B would be of much interest.

References

Borelli, D.; Fuentes, J.; Leiderman, E.; Restrepo-M.A.; Bran, J.L.; Legendre, R.; Levine, H.B. and Stevens, D.A.: Ketoconazole, an oral antifungal: laboratory and clinical assessment of imidazole drugs. Postgraduate Medical Journal 55: 657-661 (1979).

Brass, C.; Galgiani, J.N.; Campbell, S.C.; O'Reilly, R.A. and Stevens, D.A.: Therapy of coccidioidomycosis with oral ketoconazole in Nelson and Grassi (Eds) Current Chemotherapy and Infectious Disease. Vol. 2 p.965-966 (American Society for Microbiology, Washington 1980).

Conant, N.F.; Smith, D.T.; Baker, R.D. and Callaway, J.L.: Manual of Clinical Mycology, p.171-217 (Saunders, Philadelphia 1971).

DeFelice, R.; Wieden, M. and Galgiani, J.N.: Significance of Coccidioides immitis (D) in urine cultures. Presented at the 20th Interscience Conference on Antimicrobial Agents and Chemotherapy, New Orleans, Louisiana, September 22-24 (1980).

Graybill, J.R.; Lundberg, D.; Donovan, W.; Levine, H.B.; Rodriguez, M.D. and Drutz, D.J.: Treatment of coccidioidomycosis with ketoconazole: clinical and laboratory studies of 18 patients. Reviews of Infectious Diseases 2: 661-673 (1980).

Heel, R.C.; Brogden, R.N.; Pakes, G.N.; Speight, T.M. and Avery, G.S.: Miconazole: A preliminary review of its therapeutic efficacy in systemic fungal infections. Drugs 19: 7-30 (1980).

Stiller, R.L.; Defelice, R.; Brass, C.; Calgiani, J.N. and Stevens, D.A.: Therapy of cutaneous coccidioidomycosis with imidazoles. Comparison of results with miconazole and ketoconazole. Proceedings of Vth International Conference on the Mycoses, WHO Scientific Publication 396: 375-381 (1980).

Welsh, O.; Gonzalez, J.G.; Diaz, M.; Madero, D. and Gonzalez, J.: Therapeutic evaluation of ketoconazole in patients with coccidioidomycosis. Reviews of Infectious Diseases 2: 651-655 (1980).

Chapter XVIII

Subcutaneous Mycoses

(figs. 1 and 2)

The subcutaneous mycoses comprise a number of conditions including: chromomycosis (dermatitis verrucosa), eumycotic mycetoma (maduromycosis), actinomycotic mycetoma, sporotrichosis, lobomycosis (keloid blastomycosis) and rhinosporidiosis. Some of the aetiological agents in this group may not be strictly fungal; the actinomyces, for example, are higher bacteria and the agents of lobomycosis and rhinosporidosis have not been established according to Koch's postulates.

Orally administered ketoconazole has been studied in 16 patients with chromomycosis and a small number of patients with eumycotic mycetoma, actinomycotic mycetoma, sporotrichosis and lobomycosis (Borelli et al., 1979; Cuce et al., 1980; Drouhet and Dupont, 1980; unpublished data on file Janssen Research Foundation).

Open Studies in Chromomycosis

Study Methods

16 patients (1 patient was treated twice) with long-standing chromomycosis have been treated with ketoconazole. The median duration of the disease was 9 years (range 3 months to 30 years) and of the presenting episode 7.5 years. *Phialaphora* sp. was demonstrated in all patients. 7 patients had failed to respond to previous treatment with intravenously administered amphotericin B, orally administered miconazole or flucytosine or topical therapy; 8 patients had not received previous antifungal treatment.

Patients received a dose of 200 to 800mg of ketoconazole daily for a median of 14 weeks (range 4 to 29 weeks) prior to evaluation.

Results

Remission was achieved in 4 cases (24%) and marked improvement in 5 (29%). Moderate improvement occurred in 5 cases and no change was seen in 3 (table I). The median time to response was about 10 weeks (fig. 3). As shown by figure 3, the response rate may be improved with more prolonged treatment.

Increasing the daily dose of ketoconazole above 200mg did not improve the response.

Table I. Response in 17 cases (16 patients) of chromomycosis treated with orally administered ketoconazole

Clinical results	No. of cases (%)	Mycological results (%)			Serological results[1] (%)			Overall results (%)[2]			
		negative	no change	not done	negative	no change	not done	±	+	+ +	+ + +
No change	3 (18)					3 (18)					
Moderate improvement	5 (29)					5 (29)					
Marked improvement	5 (29)				2 (12)	2 (12)	1 (6)				
Clinical cure	4 (24)				2 (12)		2 (12)				
All cases	17 (100)	4 (24)	10 (59)	3 (17)	4 (24)	10 (59)	3 (18)	3 (18)	5 (29)	5 (29)	4 (24)

1 Based on specific antibodies in serum.
2 ± = no change; + = moderate improvement; + + = marked improvement; + + + = remission

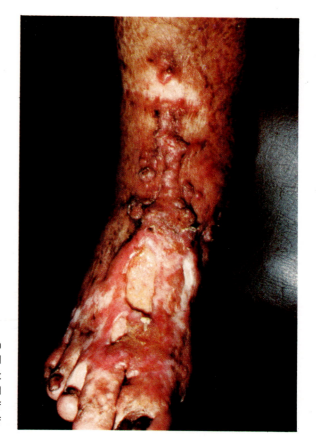

Fig. 1. A patient with chromomycosis before and after 3 months' treatment with orally administered ketoconazole. (By courtesy of Dr L.C. Cucé, University of Sao Paulo, Brazil).

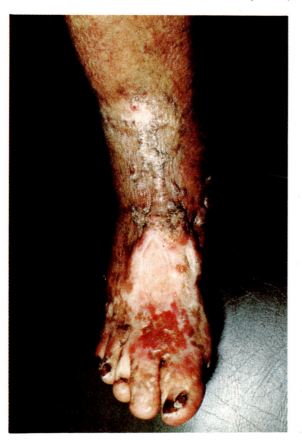

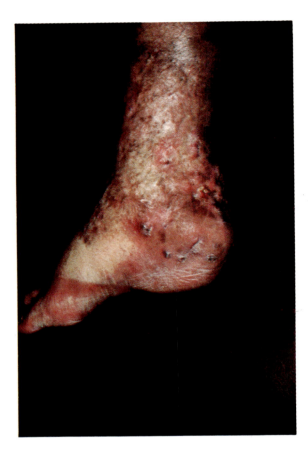

Fig. 2. Actinomycotic mycetoma before and after treatment with orally administered
ketoconazole for 5 months.
(By courtesy of Dr L.C. Cucé,
University of Sao Paulo,
Brazil).

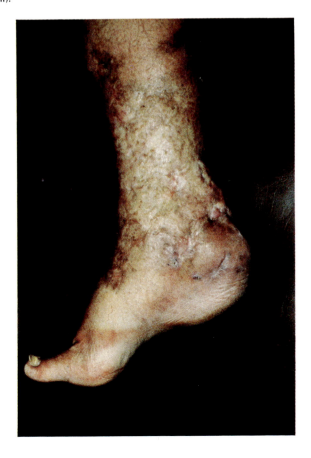

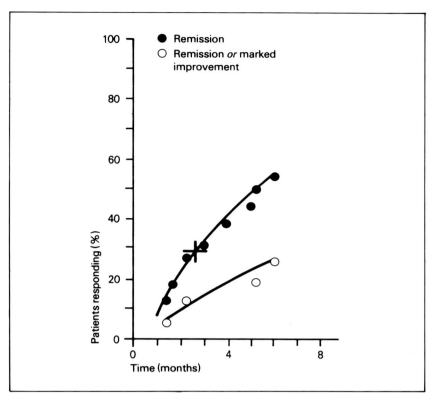

Fig. 3. Time course of response of patients with chromomycosis treated with orally administered ketoconazole. The cross indicates the median.

Other Subcutaneous Mycoses

Ketoconazole has been studied in a small number of patients with subcutaneous mycoses other than chromomycosis (table II). Although generally the numbers of patients involved are too few to make clear statements about efficacy, results in 3 patients with sporotrichosis of relatively recent onset were particularly encouraging.

Relapse

Of 4 chromomycosis patients in remission who discontinued treatment, 3 were followed for 1 to 5 months. Two patients remained in remission and the third relapsed in the fifth month after discontinuing treatment; subsequent ketoconazole treatment in this patient produced marked improvement within 1 month.

Table II. Response to treatment with orally administered ketoconazole in patients with subcutaneous mycoses other than chromomycosis

Diagnosis	No. of patients	Median duration of disease	Results[1] (%)				Time to response (+ + or + + +) in individual patients (weeks)
			±	+	+ +	+ + +	
Eumycetic mycetoma	3	19 years	1 (33)	1 (33)		1 (33)	40
Actinomycetic mycetoma	6	9 years	3 (50)	3 (50)			
Mycetoma, unspecified	2	10 years	2 (100)				
Sporotrichosis	3	10 weeks		1 (33)		2 (66)	8, 13
Lobomycosis	2	12.5 years		2 (100)			

1 ± = no change; + = moderate improvement; + + = marked improvement; + + + = remission.

Conclusions

The subcutaneous mycoses present a difficult therapeutic problem for which effective treatments have not previously been found. A response rate of 53 % in chromomycosis, as reported here with ketoconazole, may be improved upon in the future with more prolonged treatment; at the present time it represents an encouraging step forward. Further experience will be needed in other subcutaneous mycoses also before the expected response rates can be established.

References

Borelli, D.; Bran, J.L.; Fuentes, J.; Legendre, R.; Leiderman, E.; Levine, H.B.; Restrepo, A. and Stevens, D.A.: Ketoconazole, an oral antifungal: laboratory and clinical assessment of imidazole drugs. Postgraduate Medical Journal 55: 657-661 (1979).

Cuce, L.C.; Wroclawski, E.L. and Sampaio, S.A.P.: Treatment of paracoccidioidomycosis, candidosis, chromomycosis, lobomycosis, and mycetoma with ketoconazole: A brief summary. Reviews of Infectious Diseases 2: 650 (1980).

Drouhet, E. and Dupont, B.: Chronic mucocutaneous candidosis and other superficial and systemic mycoses successfully treated with ketoconazole. Reviews of Infectious Diseases 2: 606-619 (1980).

Chapter XIX

Other Areas of Use

A small number of patients with various relatively uncommon deep mycoses have been treated with orally administered ketoconazole by a number of investigators, including 7 patients with an aspergilloma, 6 patients with aspergillosis, 3 patients with cryptococcosis, 3 patients with North American blastomycosis, 2 patients with *Alternaria* infections and 1 patient each with actinomycosis, nocardiosis, chromohyphomycosis and phycomycosis (Borelli et al., 1979; Cucé et al., 1980; Drouhet and Dupont, 1980; Echenne et al., 1980; South et al., in press).

Additionally, 22 patients with advanced malignancies who were receiving cytostatic therapy have been treated with ketoconazole prophylactically for up to 1 year, and a small double-blind study has been performed in such patients.

Studies in Deep Mycoses

Study Methods

The pathogenic fungi were demonstrated in most patients; however, an *Alternaria* infection was documented historically in one patient and the diagnosis of aspergillosis was made by serology in one patient and that of aspergilloma by serology and x-ray in another patient. The diseases were relatively long-standing, with the exception of the phycomycosis infection.

Most patients were treated with a dose of 200 or 400mg of ketoconazole daily. One patient each with allergic aspergillosis and with an *Alternaria* infection were treated concomitantly with topical miconazole and one patient with phycomycosis was concurrently treated with intravenously administered amphotericin B.

Table I. Results of ketoconazole treatment in patients with miscellaneous deep mycoses

Diagnosis	No. of pts	Median duration of disease	Other concomitant treatment (no. of patients)	Results[1] (%)				Time to response (+ + or + + +) in individual patients (weeks)
				±	+	+ +	+ + +	
Aspergilloma	7	3.5 months		3 (43)	3 (43)	1 (14)		6
Aspergillosis	6[2]	8.5 months	miconazole (1)[3]	1 (17)	2 (33)	2 (33)	1 (17)	2, 3, 10
Cryptococcosis	3	6 months			1 (33)	1 (33)	1 (33)	32, 47
North American blastomycosis	3	6 months			1 (33)	1 (33)	1 (33)	20, 50
Alternaria infection	2	12 years	miconazole (1)[3]	1 (50)		1 (50)		
Actinomycosis	1	1 year		1 (100)				
Nocardiosis	1	1 year				1 (100)		45
Phycomycosis	1	1 month	amphotericin B (1)			1 (100)		5

1 ± = no change; + = moderate improvement; + + = marked improvement; + + + = remission.
2 An additional 15-year-old patient with recalcitrant disseminated aspergillosis was said to recover completely during treatment with ketoconazole 200mg daily for 4 months (Echenne et al., 1980).
3 Administered topically.

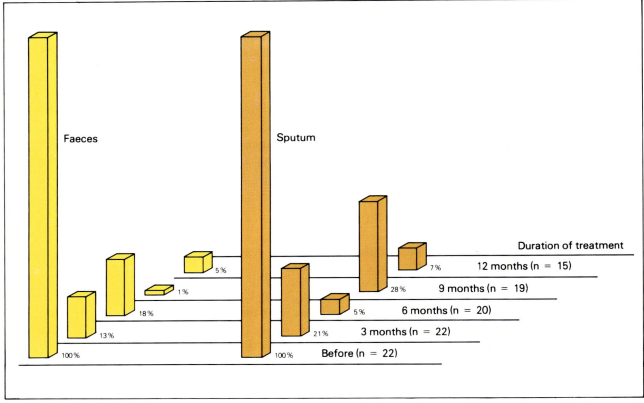

Fig. 1. Reduction in *Candida* colonisation. Relative mean concentration of *Candida* in faeces and sputum of cancer patients receiving ketoconazole 200mg daily for up to 12 months. (At the start of therapy the 100% value represents 20,000 colony forming units of *Candida* per ml in faeces and 300,000 per ml in sputum). [De Cree, personal communication.]

Results

Although the small number of patients with these various deep mycoses studied makes definitive statements about the response rates somewhat premature, results were encouraging in some conditions (table I). Some reports of individual cases studied have described the results as dramatic (e.g. Echenne et al., 1980). The accumulation of further clinical data in these areas of potential use will be awaited with interest.

Studies in the Prophylactic Use of Ketoconazole

Since patients receiving aggressive cytostatic therapy are particularly susceptible to systemic fungal infections, studies of the prophylactic use of ketoconazole in such patients are of considerable interest.

In an uncontrolled study 22 patients with advanced malignancies and receiving cytostatic therapy were treated with ketoconazole 200mg daily for up to 1 year. *Candida* in faeces and sputum was markedly suppressed during treatment, by 72 to 99% when evaluated at 3-monthly intervals (fig. 1). Of those patients with positive cultures for *Candida* prior to ketoconazole treatment, 73 to 100% improved mycologically or reverted to negative cultures. Of patients with negative cultures at the start of treatment, 80 to 100% remained negative throughout the study period.

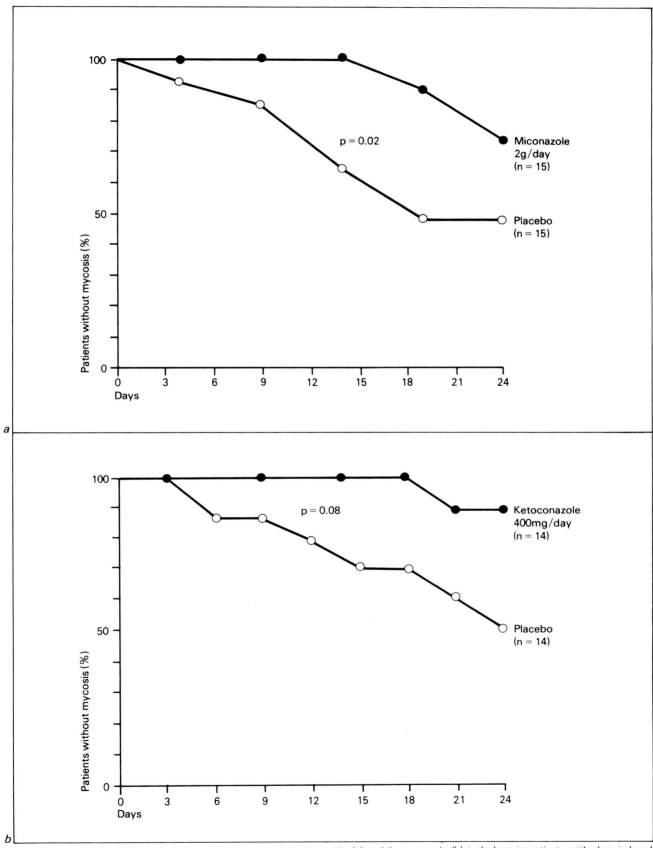

Fig. 2. The effect of prophylactic use of orally administered miconazole (a) and ketoconazole (b) in leukaemia patients with drug-induced neutropenia. (Brinker, personal communication.)

When 28 patients being treated for leukaemia received either ketoconazole 400mg daily or a placebo during the period of drug-induced neutropenia, fewer patients receiving ketoconazole developed mycoses as compared with the placebo group (fig. 2b). In a similar study using orally administered miconazole (2g daily) as the active drug (fig. 2a) results qualitatively resembled those of the ketoconazole study. Similarly, prophylactic therapy with ketoconazole 400mg daily combined with trimethoprim/sulphamethoxazole was more effective than trimethoprim/sulphamethoxazole alone in preventing febrile episodes (Maksymiuk et al., 1981). When lower doses of ketoconazole (200mg once daily) and miconazole (1g daily) were studied in like patients, disseminated candidosis was not seen at autopsy in either group, but pulmonary aspergillosis was seen in both groups (Meunier-Carpentier et al., 1981), although without a placebo or untreated control group these latter results are difficult to place in perspective.

Conclusions

In small numbers of patients with various less common deep mycoses results of ketoconazole treatment have been variable. Further clinical data will be needed to clearly establish the usefulness of the drug in these conditions. In patients undergoing cytostatic therapy the prophylactic use of ketoconazole may reduce the incidence of fungal infections.

References

Borelli, D.; Bran, J.L.; Fuentes, J.; Legendre, R.; Leiderman, E.; Levine, H.B.; Restrepo, A. and Stevens, D.A.: Ketoconazole, an oral antifungal: laboratory and clinical assessment of imidazole drugs. Postgraduate Medical Journal 55: 657-661 (1979).

Cucé, L.C.; Wrochlawski, E.L. and Sampaio, S.A.P.: Treatment of paracoccidioidomycosis, candidosis, chromomycosis, lobomycosis, and mycetoma with ketoconazole: International Journal of Dermatology 19: 405-408 (1980).

Drouhet, E. and Dupont, B.: Chronic mucocutaneous candidosis and other superficial and systemic mycoses successfully treated with ketoconazole. Reviews of Infectious Diseases 2: 606-619 (1980).

Echenne, B.; Brunel, D.; Astruc, J. and Perez, C.: Aspergillose disséminée chez un enfant porteur d'une prothèse aortique. Efficacité du ketoconazole. Médecine et Maladies Infectieuses 10: 263-266 (1980).

Maksymiuk, A.M.; Estey, E.; Keating, M.; McKelvey, E.M. and Bodey, G.P.: Infection prophylaxis during remission induction therapy in acute leukemia. American Society of Clinical Oncology, Washington, D.C., May (1981).

Meunier-Carpentier, F.; Cruciani, M. and Klastersky, J.: Antifungal prophylaxis with ketoconazole (Ke) and miconazole (Mi) in neutropenic cancer patients. International Congress of Chemotherapy, Florence, Italy, 19-24 July (1981).

Samelson, L.E.; Lerner, S.A.; Resnekov, L. and Anagnostopoulos, C.: Relapse of *Candida parapsilosis* endocarditis after long-term suppression with flucytosine: retreatment with valve replacement and ketoconazole. Annals of Internal Medicine 93: 838-839 (1980).

South, D.A.; Brass, C. and Stephens, D.A.: Chromohyphomycosis: Treatment with ketoconazole. Archives of Dermatology (in press).

Weisburd, G.J. and Bonazzola, R.: R41400, ketoconazole, en el tratamiento de las micosis profundas. IX Jornadas Argentinas de Micologia, Resistencia, Chaco, Rep. Argentina July 31-August 4 (1979).

Practical Aspects of Treatment

Chapter XX

Practical Clinical Considerations

Dosage and Administration

Dosage Schedules

The majority of adult patients studied so far have received a single daily dose of ketoconazole 200mg (given orally), which was arrived at empirically based on pharmacokinetic and pharmacodynamic data, toxicity studies and early clinical experience. This is the initial dosage schedule recommended for all conditions, with the exception of vaginal candidosis. In this condition the preferred dosage schedule is related to the need for a total dose of at least 1200mg; a dose of 200mg given twice daily for 5 days is the dose recommended by the manufacturers. In all conditions, if the clinical response is inadequate at the initial dosage level, the dose may be increased to 400 or 600mg once daily; however, at present there is little evidence to support an improved response with higher doses.

Up to mid-1980 a small number of children, including some infants, had been treated with ketoconazole. More than 175 patients less than 15 years of age have been treated. On the basis of this data the recommended dosage schedule in children is as follows:

  i) children weighing 20kg or less: 50mg once daily
 ii) children weighing more than 20 and up to 40kg: 100mg once daily
iii) children weighing more than 40kg: 200mg once daily.

A suspension dosage form (20mg/ml) of the drug is at present being developed to facilitate administration in young children or in others who cannot readily swallow a tablet. Most children will thus receive 1ml of this dose form 3 times a day, based on their body weight.

Table I. General guidelines for the duration of ketoconazole treatment in patients with fungal infections

Condition	Usual treatment period[1]
Superficial mycoses	
Dermatomycoses	4-8 weeks
Hair or scalp mycoses	4-8 weeks
Pityriasis versicolor	3-6 weeks
Oral thrush	1-2 weeks
Vaginal candidosis	5 days
Chronic mucocutaneous candidosis	6-12 months
Onychomycosis	6-12 months
Deep mycoses[2]	
Systemic candidosis	2-4 weeks
Candiduria	2-4 weeks
Paracoccidioidomycosis	2-4 months
Coccidioidomycosis	> 6 months
Histoplasmosis	2-4 months
Chromomycosis	> 6 months

1   The final decision in individual patients should be based on clinical and mycological response whenever possible. Continued prophylactic use to prevent relapse is probably justified in some patients (see text).
2   In deep mycoses treatment should continue for at least 1 week after apparent eradication of the infecting fungus.

In all patients the drug should be taken with a meal, and concomitant therapy with agents which reduce gastric acidity should be avoided (see chapter VI). If therapy with drugs such as antacids, anticholinergics or histamine H_2-blockers such as cimetidine is considered necessary they should be given at least 2 hours after ketoconazole.

Duration of Treatment

The duration of treatment in patients with fungal infections should be based on the clinical and mycological responses, and thus must be individualised. General guidelines for suggested periods of treatment with ketoconazole are shown in table I.

Relapse is a common problem in many fungal infections, and continued prophylactic use of ketoconazole to prevent relapse is probably justified for certain time periods in some patients. However, this is an area in which only scant data are available at present; further studies are needed to clarify the merits of using ketoconazole in this way, the optimum dosage for prophylactic use and the most suitable duration of prophylactic therapy in various conditions.

Table II. Response to ketoconazole therapy in various sub-groups of patients with mycoses compared with the response in patients in whom the particular factor did not apply

Sub-group of patients	Response					
	superficial mycoses			deep mycoses		
	no. of patients	patients in sub-group %	patients not in sub-group %	no. of patients	patients in sub-group %	patients not in sub-group %
Antacid therapy	3	67	87	13	38[1]	65[1]
Antibiotic therapy	25	76	87	84	69	62
Corticosteroid therapy	58	86	87	33	70	63
Immunodeficiency	34	63[2]	88[2]	17	53	65
Diabetes mellitus	12	83	87	33	24[3]	69[3]
Thyroid dysfunction	15	47[2]	87[2]	6	67	64
Addison's disease	5	80	87	4	100	64
Neoplasms	13	77	87	12	58	64
Catheters/prostheses				15	67	64
Renal failure	1	100	87	17	59	64
No response to antifungal treatment	310	86	88[4]	30	80	88[4]

1   $p = 0.09$.
2   $p < 0.01$.
3   $p < 0.0001$.
4   Response in patients with no previous antifungal treatment.

Factors Influencing Response

As discussed in individual chapters there were few occasions when particular patient's characteristics or other aspects of treatment, such as dosage, duration of disease, etc., could be clearly correlated with the response to ketoconazole. In many instances there were probably insufficient numbers of patients in the various sub-groups to clearly establish a correlation with response if any existed. Pooling such data suggests that patients with immunodeficiency, diabetes mellitus, thyroid dysfunction or those receiving antacid therapy may be less likely to respond than others (table II).

Side Effects

Ketoconazole has been well tolerated in most patients. In a survey of 1361 patients, 199 (17%) reported side effects (table III) — most frequently nausea/vomiting (3%), pruritus (1.7%) or abdominal pain (1.3%). All other reported reactions occurred with a frequency of less than 1%. Many of the symptoms shown in the table occurred in single instances only; their association with ketoconazole administration is, of course, open to question, especially since patients often were receiving concomitant therapy. The dosage of ketoconazole was reduced because of side effects in 8 patients (0.7%), or 4% of those reporting side effects. Ketoconazole treatment was discontinued because of side effects in 17 patients (1.5%) permanently and in 15 patients (1.3%) temporarily, or in 8.5% and 7.5% respectively of patients reporting side effects.

Table III. Side effects reported during ketoconazole treatment in 1361 adult patients with fungal infections

Reported side effects	Incidence (%)	Concomitant treatment[1]	Ketoconazole discontinued[1,2]	Ketoconazole dosage reduced[1]
Gastrointestinal effects				
Nausea/vomiting	3	18/38	8/38	5/38
Abdominal pain	1.3	4/16	2/16	1/16
Diarrhoea	0.7	2/8		
'GI disorder'	0.4	2/5		
Dyspepsia	0.2			
Flatulence	0.1			
Discoloration of tongue	0.1			
Gastrointestinal bleeding	0.1			
Dermatological effects				
Pruritus	1.7	9/20	1/20	1/20
Rash	0.7	4/8	3/8	
Dermatitis	0.2	1/2		
Changes in sweat pattern	0.2	1/2		
Alopecia	0.2	2/2		
Photosensitivity	0.1	1/1		
Burning sensation	0.1	1/1		
Purpura	0.1			
Musculoskeletal and nervous system effects				
Dizziness	0.8	4/9	1/9	
Somnolence	0.8	4/9	2/9	
Asthenia	0.3	3/4	1/4	
Arthralgia	0.3	2/4		
Myalgia	0.3	2/3	1/3	
Insomnia	0.2			
Nervousness	0.2	1/2	1/2	
Abnormal dreams	0.1			
Paraesthesia	0.1	1/1		

(continued on next page)

(continued from previous page)

Reported side effects	Incidence (%)	Concomitant treatment[1]	Ketoconazole discontinued[1,2]	Ketoconazole dosage reduced[1]
Metabolic and nutritional effects				
Increased alkaline phosphatase	0.3	1/4		
Increased SGOT	0.1		1/1	
Hyperlipidaemia	0.3			
Anorexia	0.2	1/2		
Increased appetite	0.1			
Weight gain	0.1		1/1	
Increased SGPT	0.1		1/1	
Acidosis	0.1	1/1		
Avitaminosis D	0.1	1/1		
Hyperbilirubinaemia	0.1			
Ocular effects				
Photophobia	0.2	2/2		
Blepharitis	0.1	1/1	1/1	
Visual acuity disorder	0.1		1/1	
Retinal disorder	0.1			
Cardiovascular effects				
Hypertension	0.1		1/1	
Palpitations	0.1			
Thrombophlebitis	0.1	1/1		
Vasodilation	0.1	1/1		
Effects on the haematopoietic/lymphatic systems				
Decreased haematocrit	0.1	1/1		
Thrombocytopenia	0.1	1/1		
Eosinophilia	0.1	1/1		
Leukopenia/neutropenia	0.1	1/1		
Miscellaneous				
Headache	0.9	3/10		
Fever/chills	0.3	2/3	2/3	
Gynaecomastia	0.2			
Malaise	0.1			
Epistaxis	0.1	1/1		
Impotence	0.1	1/1		
Alcohol intolerance	0.1			
'Bad' taste	0.1	1/1		
Otitis media	0.1		1/1	

1   Number of patients receiving concomitant treatment, or in whom ketoconazole was discontinued or the dosage reduced because of side effects/total number of patients reporting that side effect.

2   Permanent or temporary discontinuation of treatment; in some patients ketoconazole treatment was discontinued for a short period and then re-instituted.

In children ketoconazole appears to be particularly well tolerated. Adverse effects occurred in 2 of 62 patients up to 5 years of age: transient fever and chills in a 3-year-old child receiving a dose of 7.7mg/kg, and persistent gastrointestinal upset (diarrhoea, nausea and vomiting) in a 5-year-old receiving 6.7 to 13.3mg/kg. In the latter case treatment was discontinued.

Chapter XXI

Ketoconazole in Perspective

Drugs Available for Superficial Mycoses

It is always a difficult task to place a new drug into proper perspective, defining its role in therapy. An attempt to do so must be preceded by an understanding of the relative merits and shortcomings of other similar agents, and must inevitably be accompanied by a discussion of those areas in which further study with the new drug is needed.

Many topical antifungal drugs are available for the treatment of superficial mycoses; some such agents, particularly those developed relatively recently such as nystatin, clotrimazole, econazole, miconazole etc. represent effective therapy for certain superficial infections if used correctly. However, topical therapy is often inconvenient or 'messy', and as a result may be particularly susceptible to non-compliance by patients. (In the case of vaginal candidosis this has been partially but not completely overcome by recently introduced 'short term' treatment regimens with some topical preparations). Griseofulvin (p.16) is an effective drug for dermatophytic infections at sites where new keratin is being formed although infections of the nails, toe webs or inflamed areas may respond less readily (Marks, 1980). Although generally a 'safe' drug, side effects (headache, gastrointestinal upset, photosensitivity) can be troublesome in some patients. Thus, an effective and safe orally administered agent with a wide spectrum of antifungal activity for treatment of superficial fungal infections is an exciting consideration.

Drugs Available for Deep Mycoses

The drugs available for the chemotherapy of systemic fungal infections have recently been the subject of concise reviews (Medoff and Kobayashi, 1980; Utz, 1980).

Potassium iodide is effective in treating sporotrichosis (more so in the cutaneous-lymphatic form than in other forms of the disease), but iodism is frequently encountered. Other fungal infections, possibly excepting infection with *Basidiobolus haptosporus,* do not reliably respond to treatment with iodides.

Hydroxystilbamidine isethionate must be given by daily intravenous infusion over the course of several weeks (see chapter II). Its relative effectiveness in blastomycosis (its only important area of potential usefulness in fungal infections) is still a matter of some controversy. It is usually recommended that it be reserved for nonprogressive cutaneous forms of the disease.

Amphotericin B has a relatively wide range of antifungal activity *in vitro* and has been used in many types of fungal infection (see chapter II). It has been most useful in progressive blastomycosis, histoplasmosis, cryptococcal infections, paracoccidioidomycosis, severe sporotrichosis and chromomycosis. Its usefulness in coccidioidomycosis, severe systemic candidosis, phycomycoses and *Aspergillus* infections is more limited. Amphotericin B suffers from the disadvantages of requiring parenteral administration and potentially serious side effects, either or both of which may make treatment for an adequate period of time difficult. Renal toxicity occurs frequently, and azotaemia is often a dose limiting factor. Hypokalaemia, with resultant cardiac arrhythmias and muscular weakness if uncorrected, occurs in about 25% of patients. Leukopenia and thrombocytopenia occur less frequently. Cerebrospinal fluid concentrations of the drug are much lower than plasma concentrations, often necessitating intrathecal administration in fungal meningitis; as with intravenous administration, side effects are frequently a limiting factor with intrathecal therapy.

Flucytosine, which can be given orally and reaches cerebrospinal fluid more readily than amphotericin B, avoids the administration difficulties of amphotericin B, and is relatively well tolerated, but it has a narrow spectrum of useful activity (*Cryptococcus neoformans* and species of *Candida, Torulopsis* and the agents of chromomycosis) limiting its therapeutic potential. Even in these groups of fungi marked variation in sensitivity may occur and resistance is a problem (p.16).

Miconazole, a broad spectrum antifungal imidazole like ketoconazole, may be useful in some patients with systemic or mucocutaneous candidosis, coccidioidomycosis, paracoccidioidomycosis or cryptococcal infections (Heel et al., 1980), but clinical experience is limited in most areas. Miconazole is poorly absorbed from the gastrointestinal tract, requiring parenteral administration in most situations. Side effects, which can be troublesome include phlebitis, pruritus, nausea, fever or chills and rash.

Thus, it is apparent that all of the drugs at present available for treating systemic fungal infections have important shortcomings. How does ketoconazole 'measure up' in comparison?

Ketoconazole: Its Place in Therapy

At the onset it must be understood that the place of ketoconazole in the therapy of fungal disease cannot yet be definitively described; it is still relatively early in the clinical development of this agent and further study is needed in a number of areas. The following points must be kept in mind.

i) In most fungal conditions the number of patients studied is small, suggesting that particular caution is needed in interpreting the data.
ii) Ketoconazole has not been studied in a sufficient number of patients with fungal meningitis. Although potentially useful cerebrospinal fluid concentrations occurred in a few patients after oral administration of the drug, CSF concentrations are lower than serum concentrations; it is unclear if orally administered ketoconazole alone is appropriate in fungal meningitis.
iii) A proportion of the patients discussed in preceding chapters were still being treated at the time of evaluation, so that the final response rates could ultimately vary from those reported.
iv) A third of the patients studied had failed to respond to previous antifungal treatment and thus could be considered as presenting an especial therapeutic challenge.
v) Only a very small number of patients in ketoconazole-induced remission have been followed-up; in the few who were followed the duration of follow-up was often inadequate to clearly establish the relapse rate.
vi) There is as yet little experience with long-term administration of ketoconazole in chronic conditions and/or to prevent relapse.
vii) A particular difficulty in evaluating the relative efficacy of ketoconazole is the uncontrolled nature of most of the data available. With the exception of a few small controlled studies in superficial mycoses, no comparative studies have been performed. A small number of well designed

comparative studies, for example using amphotericin B as the comparative drug in deep mycoses in which it has proved useful, and griseofulvin in dermatophyte infections of the skin and nails, would do much to overcome this problem.

Despite these cautionary notes it can be said that ketoconazole is an exciting new development. It has a broad spectrum of antifungal activity including useful *in vivo* activity against most common pathogenic fungi, it is absorbed from the gastrointestinal tract sufficiently well to allow oral therapy, and some aspects of its distribution profile (e.g. probable passage into sebum) make it particularly suitable for treating superficial mycoses (although as stated above its passage into cerebrospinal fluid needs further clarification). It appears to be well tolerated, keeping in mind the limited long-term experience. Based on the clinical efficacy so far demonstrated, ketoconazole seems to offer most potential usefulness in dermatomycoses, pityriasis versicolor, oral and vaginal candidal infections, paracoccidioidomycosis, histoplasmosis, mycoses of the scalp, hair or nails and chronic mucocutaneous candidosis, with moderate effectiveness coccidioidomycosis and chromomycosis. In the few patients studied its usefulness in *Aspergillus* infections has been variable, ranging from ineffectiveness in some to apparently outstanding effectiveness in others.

Conclusion

The concept of an effective and safe orally absorbed broad spectrum antifungal drug must capture the imagination of all involved in the difficult therapeutic area of fungal disease. Although it is too early in the drug's clinical life to state clearly the ultimate place of ketoconazole in the treatment of fungal diseases, the drug represents a major important advance in antifungal chemotherapy. Ketoconazole may well become the 'drug of choice' in many mycotic diseases.

References

Heel, R.C.; Brogden, R.N.; Pakes, G.E.; Speight, T.M. and Avery, G.S.: Miconazole: a preliminary review of its therapeutic efficacy in systemic fungal infections. Drugs 19: 7-30 (1980).

Marks, J.: Skin Diseases; in Avery (Ed) Drug Treatment 2nd Edition, p.335 (Churchill Livingstone, Edinburgh; Adis Press, Sydney 1980).

Medoff, G. and Kobayashi, G.S.: Strategies in the treatment of systemic fungal infections. New England Journal of Medicine 302: 145-155 (1980).

Utz, J.P.: Chemotherapy for systemic mycoses: the prelude to ketoconazole. Reviews of Infectious Diseases 2: 625-632 (1980).

Subject Index